EVERYD
HOMOEOPA

A Safe Guide For Self Treatment

SECOND EDITION

Dr David M. Gemmell
MB, BS, BSc, MFHom

BEACONSFIELD PUBLISHERS LTD
Beaconsfield, Bucks, UK

First published in 1987
Second edition 1997

British Library Cataloguing in Publication Data
Gemmell, David M.
Everyday homoeopathy. – 2nd ed. –
(Beaconsfield homoeopathic library; no. 17)
1. Homeopathy
I. Title
615.5'32

ISBN 0–906584–44–2

Phototypeset by Gem Graphics, Trenance, Mawgan Porth, Cornwall,
in 10 on 12 point Times
Printed in Great Britain at The Bath Press, Bath

Acknowledgements

I owe a great deal to my wife, Irma, for her encouragement. Our discussions about the design of the book and her editing of the various sections contributed much to its final form.

David Gemmell

Note

Mrs Irma Gemmell and the Publisher are sad to record that Dr David Gemmell died before being able to complete his preparation of this Second Edition. We would like to express our warm appreciation to Dr Janet Gray for continuing the work and bringing the manuscript into its present form for publication. We would also like to record our thanks to Dr Alice Greene for valuable comments she provided at the outset of the revision and which Dr Gemmell was pleased to be able to take into account.

Contents

Contents

Introduction

Why this Book has been Written

Increasing numbers of people are becoming anxious about the severe toxic effects of many modern drugs. There is also great concern about the problem of addiction to prescribed tranquillisers, sedatives and pain-killers. Examples of such problems are almost certainly familiar to each of us.

Parents have become alarmed at the way that small children with recurring ear, nose and throat infections, and chest infections, are prescribed course after course of potent antibiotics. Catarrh is 'dried up' with drugs which at the same time not infrequently cause some degree of hyperactivity and sleeplessness. Older men may find that they have exchanged symptomless high blood pressure for a life of malaise, cold hands and feet, and impotence. Others will discover that the price of fast relief from the pain of rheumatism is severe indigestion, and occasionally ulceration and bleeding.

With all these problems there is a widespread feeling that we have handed ourselves over to 'the experts' – that we have lost the ability to participate in healing ourselves.

The development of modern scientific medicine has unquestionably brought enormous benefits to millions of people. But the price of overuse has often been the alienation of the individual patient from the medical profession, which, for its part, has been overwhelmed by the endless demands made upon it. People are also rediscovering that to acquire good health, and maintain it, they must begin to take responsibility for themselves and their families: 'You are part of the healing team – not a puppet or inert object of medical or surgical techniques. It is essential that you participate in your own recovery.' (Quoted from *Healing for Everyone – Medicine of the Whole Person*, by E. G. Loomis and J. S. Paulson, De Vorss Publishing Co., Marina del Rey, California, USA.)

The first step towards acquiring and maintaining good health can only be taken by positive attention to diet, appropriate exercise, rest and relaxation, and the development of emotional and spiritual maturity.

The second step is to avoid the over-use of alcohol, as well as any use of tobacco and other drugs of addiction.

The third step is to appreciate that some illness is an inevitable part of life itself. Illness often indicates a lack of harmony in life as a whole.

The re-establishing of harmony may be achieved by attention to lifestyle, both short- and long-term, and by the use of various gentle and non-invasive therapies.

This is where homoeopathic medicine comes in.

Homoeopathic medicine works at different levels. It can be used by anyone for minor or short-lived health problems, even with limited knowledge or advice. At its most sophisticated, homoeopathy acts on the whole person and requires deep knowledge and much experience.

Homoeopathy provides a safe, inexpensive and frequently speedy method of treatment which can be used either in its own right or before turning to the more conventional treatments. It can be used on its own, or *in conjunction with* orthodox treatments. Homoeopathic medicine is complementary to all other forms of treatment.

This book is intended to help you and your family to use homoeopathy, at home and in safety. The problems I discuss are suitable for treatment by the reader. Wherever I feel it is essential to obtain professional advice, either initially or later on, this has been indicated.

If it is used as intended for minor health problems, you will almost certainly find that you need to call upon your own doctor's services less frequently. The fact that you have used homoeopathic remedies need concern him or her no more than if you had used any other self-help method.

It is important that you should have a National Health Service general practitioner, because sooner or later there will be a situation which will need orthodox treatment – such as surgery, accident care, expensive investigations or long-term support.

Take care to maintain the sympathy and concern of your general practitioner by not demanding too aggressively that he or she becomes convinced of the effectiveness of homoeopathic medicine. It is a free country and doctors are as entitled to their own opinions as you are to yours.

Difficulties may arise when you ask to be referred to a homoeopathic doctor, or else to a homoeopathic consultant physician at one of the National Health Service homoeopathic hospitals (see page 215). This usually arises when all orthodox approaches to a problem have failed. You may suggest a second opinion, and if you wish that it should be from a homoeopathic physician, then that facility is available to you under the NHS. But please be diplomatic in making your request.

Homoeopathic doctors have always worked within the traditional ethical framework of the medical profession, but have sometimes been frustrated by the reactions engendered in their orthodox colleagues by undiplomatic patients. Many general practitioners have recently become much more accepting of homoeopathic medicine, and it would be a pity to antagonise them with overenthusiastic or unrealistic expectations.

What is Homoeopathy?

Homoeopathy is a system of medical treatment using medicine according to the principle of 'like cures like'.

As a theory and a means of treatment it was taught in Hindu writings over three thousand years ago. It was mentioned in the writings of Hippocrates in Ancient Greece. Galen described it in the second century in Rome. Paracelsus, the famous alchemist-physician, practised it in sixteenth-century Europe. Throughout this long history the emphasis and sophistication have changed, but the principle has remained the same.

The principle is based on the observation that substances which cause symptoms can also be used to cure them. The homoeopathic method attempts to match the symptoms of a sick person with the description of the toxic effects of a particular substance. The same substance, in a much diluted form, can then be safely used as a medicine for the sick person.

It was a German physician, Samuel Hahnemann, who rediscovered the principle of homoeopathy around the year 1800. Hahnemann was one of the first doctors to research into the medicine of his day, using himself, his family and his students as guinea-pigs. The following facts emerged from his work:

- Overdoses of the common medicines then in use caused side effects which could be recognised as distinct patterns of poisoning.
- Patients reacting individually to disease developed particular patterns of illness.
- It was often possible to match the pattern of the patient's illness with the pattern of the drug overdose observed in his experiments.

The next step was to treat the patient with the correctly matched drug, and note the frequency of successful treatment. Because of the strength of the doses that were then considered necessary, patients very often became worse before getting better. So Hahnemann diluted his medicines by stages in an alcohol and water solution, giving them a vigorous mechanical shaking (termed 'succussion') between each stage of dilution. He discovered that these medicines were as effective as the concentrated ones but did not give rise to toxic effects. He also found that medicines prepared in this way remained medically active for several years.

Hahnemann experimented with the effects of many of the medicines of the time, such as quinine, and he also discovered the medicinal qualities of many new substances such as gold and silver. His successors in homoeopathy have continued to explore the use of many more substances, so that by now there are nearly three thousand of them. However, this little book is only concerned with about thirty remedies, because experience has shown that most common family illnesses can be helped by them.

Many examples of the homoeopathic principle in treatment are found in modern 'scientific medicine'. Generally they are unrecognised by patients as well as by the orthodox doctors who use them. For instance, X-ray overdosage can cause some types of cancer, whereas carefully controlled doses of X-rays can also cure some types of cancer. Amphetamines normally cause nervous excitability and physical overactivity, but a dramatic effect can be seen in the use of amphetamines for calming some hyperactive children.

How to Use this Book

1) Look up the section you need (e.g. 'The Baby', page 70). Alternatively, check the Problem Index at the end of the book for the page number of your problem.
2) Turn to the appropriate page and read the left-hand page for the background information (e.g. 'Feeding Problems').
3) Read the right-hand page for the short description of the symptoms (e.g. 'Wind and Colic').
4) Compare these descriptions with the symptoms of the patient, and select the one which is the most similar (e.g. 'Chilly, irritable, angry. Overfeeding').
5) Read off the name of the remedy suggested at the right of the chosen symptom description, together with the potency and the dosage scheme (e.g. '**Nux Vomica 6c**. One dose every half hour for up to 3 doses. Repeat when necessary.').

How to Select the Symptoms

As you use this book you will become aware that homoeopathic medicine aims to treat the patient as an individual and as a whole. What marks him as an individual is his own 'symptom picture'. The things which make his symptom picture unique are his personal reactions to conditions like the weather, the seasons, the time of day or the way he is affected by movement or rest. His emotional make-up is most important too.

The Remedy

You will notice that some remedies will be suggested for several different and apparently unrelated conditions. This is because these homoeopathic remedies affect the living processes in every part of the body and so are found to be medically active in many conditions. In other words, these major remedies are medicines for the whole person.

While it is important to take all the symptoms of a patient into account, this may in practice not always be possible: the purpose of this book is to show how even a limited view of the patient can help you to choose an effective remedy.

The remedies may be bought as pills, tablets, powders or granules. They are all made of lactose (milk sugar) and they have all been medicated in the same way with the liquid form of the remedy. The actual form makes no difference. Tablets are most commonly available: some may be harder than others and take longer to dissolve.

While pills and tablets are convenient for children and adults, powders are more suitable for babies. If powders of a remedy are not available, a tablet or a pill can be crushed between two clean, dry teaspoons.

Certain remedies are used in ointments or creams, and can be bought directly from chemists and health food shops. These remedies can also be used in solutions, and in this case are sold as alcoholic tinctures to be used either neat or else diluted with water.

When a tincture is to be diluted, we suggest you use 5ml of tincture in 200ml of cool, previously boiled water. If you find the pint measure more convenient, 20 drops of tincture in half a pint of cool, previously boiled water is more or less equivalent. These ratios are meant to be a rule-of-thumb, and do not need to be followed precisely.

Do not treat yourself with homoeopathic remedies if you are already being treated by a homoeopath. Check with him or her first unless the new condition is a simple one, such as using Arnica for bruising in a minor injury.

The Dose

In homoeopathic medicine it is not possible to be dogmatic about dosage and prescribing methods, because they are adjusted to each individual patient and his changing symptoms. Adjustments may have to be made following each change of symptoms.

One dose of a remedy consists of one pill, or one tablet, or one powder, or ten to fifteen granules.

Some manufacturers suggest giving one tablet for a child and two for an adult. Strictly speaking, one tablet is all that is necessary for either a child or an adult, but if in doubt, follow the suggestions on the container.

Remember that the recommended doses are only a guide and that with practice you will develop confidence in your own judgement.

Continuing the Dose

Several doses of a remedy may be needed before improvement occurs. The dosage scheme under the name of the chosen remedy on the right of the right-hand page will indicate the sort of timing likely to be needed. But remember that every case is different, so give the remedy more or less frequently depending on the response of the patient.

It is safe to give some remedies as frequently as every ten minutes. It is more common to give a remedy two, three or four times a day. *Whatever the circumstances, it is important that the remedy should be discontinued as soon as there is an improvement in the condition.* If you carry on for longer than is necessary you may provoke a resurgence of the original symptoms or else cause new ones to arise. (If this does happen, stop the remedy and wait for the new symptoms to subside, and then reassess the situation.)

It is difficult to be dogmatic about how long to take a remedy, since every patient is different. Usually long-term illness takes longer to treat, and short-term illness responds to treatment more quickly. But there will be exceptions. If the condition does not respond after following the dosage instructions provided, it is probable that the wrong remedy has been chosen, and it should be stopped. In this case, read the description of the symptoms again, and observe any *changes* in symptoms or *new* symptoms which may have developed in the patient. Change the remedy to suit the new symptoms.

If the original symptoms become worse, *stop taking the remedy*. This may be what homoeopaths call an 'aggravation' of symptoms and is generally a good omen. The problem is likely to get better on its own without further treatment. Later, if the same symptoms recur, take the remedy again but less often than before.

Homoeopathy is a very practical system of treatment. If the patient does not improve after using your second choice of remedy, **do not** press on regardless. The wellbeing of the patient is paramount, and no one should be trying to prove anything. There are occasions when other help is needed, and you should reconsider the condition of the patient. If you are in any doubt, consult a homoeopath or your own family practitioner.

Potency

The potency of a remedy is a very precise concept. It refers to the extent and the number of times the original extract of the remedy has been diluted during the preparation. As an example, Arnica 6c has been prepared as follows:

One drop of the original alcoholic extract of the Arnica plant is added to 99 drops of a solution of water and alcohol, and shaken or vibrated vigorously (in the process mentioned earlier as 'succussion'). This diluted solution is known as the first centesimal potency of Arnica, or Arnica 1c.

One drop of this new solution (1c) is diluted again in a further 99 drops of the solution of water and alcohol, shaken vigorously and so becomes the second potency (Arnica 2c).

One drop of this latest solution (2c) is added to a further 99 drops of the water and alcohol solution, vigorously shaken and this becomes the third potency (Arnica 3c).

This process of serial dilution and succussion continues through the stages to Arnica 6c. In practice any number of dilutions can be made.

It is in these repeated stages of 'potentisation' that the original substance is diluted to the point where the risk of any side effect is eliminated. At the same time the therapeutic effectiveness of the substance is either greatly enhanced or else first becomes apparent.

The potency usually referred to in this book is 6c. It is used here because it is highly effective and also because it is the one that is most commonly available in shops in the United Kingdom.

As a rough guide, the 6c potency is used for conditions which are mainly physical, for example bruising, rheumatism or hay fever. This potency would tend to be repeated frequently, say every two hours for a day or so in the case of bruising, or three times a day for a few days for painful joints.

A more experienced prescriber may wish to give a 30c potency when the condition affects the patient more generally. The 30c potency tends to be used for illnesses which may be partly emotional in nature, such as anxiety before examinations, sleeplessness or even acute bronchitis. A few doses at intervals of every four or six hours is often all that is needed, although the effects of a nervous shock might need a few doses of a 30c every half hour or so.

Remedies in the 30c potency can be obtained either in person or by post from chemists who stock homoeopathic remedies. A current list of homoeopathic pharmacies is available from any of the organisations shown on pages 216–17. There are many 'higher' potencies available in homoeopathy; that is, the remedies have been diluted and succussed many times more than the 30c potency. They should only be used by an experienced homoeopath and not by the home prescriber.

It is quite possible that you will also come across remedies in the 'x' or 'decimal' potency. These are prepared in a ratio of 1 to 9 drops instead of the 1 to 99 drops of the 'c' potency.

If you wish to prescribe a remedy but the available potency is different from the one suggested in the book, do not despair or give up. *Use the potency that you have*. It is important to remember that the fundamental reason for prescribing a particular remedy is *the similarity of the symptoms of the patient with the symptom picture of the remedy*. In principle the potency is less important than the correct choice of the remedy.

Important Points to Remember about Homoeopathic Remedies

- Remedies should be placed on the tongue and allowed to dissolve. *Do not* take with food and *do not* wash down with a drink.
- Allow about twenty minutes before or after anything else is put into the mouth. That includes foods, drinks, toothpaste, tobacco and other medicines.
- Remedies can be given in complete safety to old people, children and babies.
- They are pleasant to taste and so are popular with children.
- They are *not* poisonous. However, remember that *all* medicines, including homoeopathic ones, should be kept out of reach of children.
- They can be used in pregnancy with complete safety.
- They do not interfere with ordinary medicine, which can continue to be taken if necessary. But do not take them simultaneously. If at all possible, you should allow about twenty minutes between different medicines.
- They will be inactivated if spilled, handled more than necessary, over-heated, exposed to sunlight or otherwise contaminated.
- They should be stored away from light at normal room temperatures, and away from strong-smelling substances such as scent, aromatherapy oils, antiseptics, liniments, vapour rubs, mothballs and so on.
- The containers should be kept tightly sealed. If the remedies are kept in glass bottles they will remain active for several years. It is not known how long remedies in the new, plastic containers will remain effective. Experience suggests that it is over two years.

ACCIDENTS AND FIRST AID

Note: If you need to take someone to the Accident & Emergency Department of a hospital (also called A&E or Casualty Department), it is essential that you check first where this is. Not every hospital has an A&E Department. You will find the numbers in the phone book under 'Hospitals'.

ANIMAL BITES

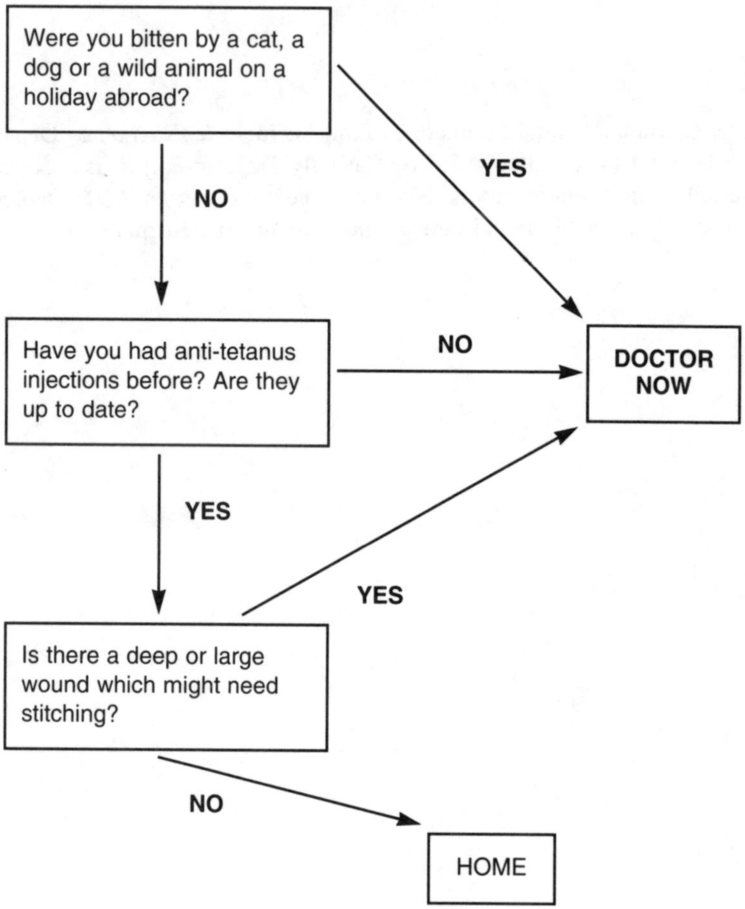

ANIMAL BITES

Small bites can easily be treated at home.

By Mouth

For pain, especially in very sensitive areas, e.g. fingertips. Alternate with Calendula, if you feel that both are needed.	**Hypericum 6c.** One three times a day for 2–3 days.
To reduce infection and promote healing.	**Ledum 6c** and **Calendula 6c.** One dose every fifteen minutes for the first hour. Then take one three times a day for 3–5 days.

Application to the Bite

Clean the wound with warm soap and water. Bathe with a freshly prepared solution of **Calendula** or **Hypercal**. This is made by adding 5ml (20 drops) of the tincture to 200ml (half a pint) of cool, previously boiled, water. Use fresh solutions for each bathing. Dress the wound with a sterile, unmedicated dressing kept moistened with the Calendula or Hypercal solution.

BURNS AND SCALDS

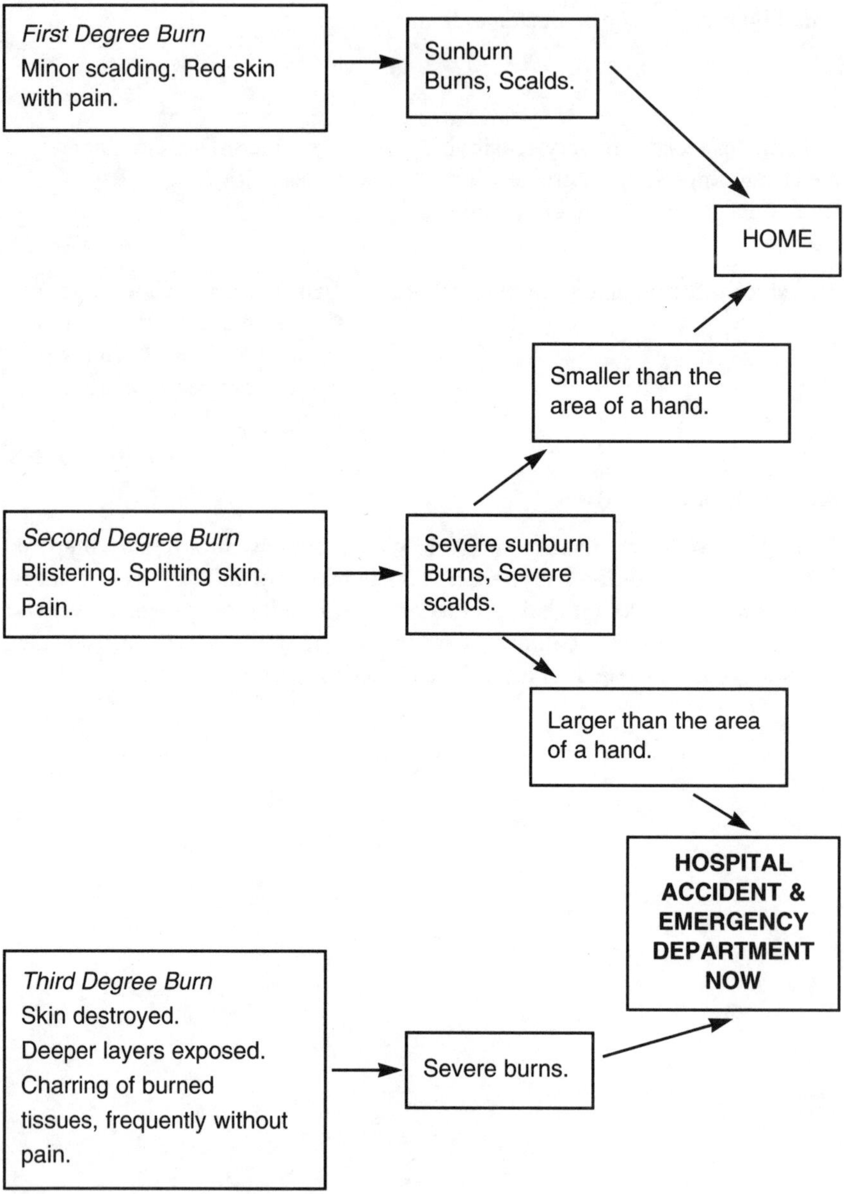
First Degree Burn
Minor scalding. Red skin with pain.
Sunburn
Burns, Scalds.
HOME
Smaller than the area of a hand.
Second Degree Burn
Blistering. Splitting skin. Pain.
Severe sunburn
Burns, Severe scalds.
Larger than the area of a hand.
HOSPITAL ACCIDENT & EMERGENCY DEPARTMENT NOW
Third Degree Burn
Skin destroyed.
Deeper layers exposed.
Charring of burned tissues, frequently without pain.
Severe burns.

BURNS AND SCALDS

Immediate First Aid

Immerse in cold water for five to ten minutes.

Application to the Burn or Scald

Apply sterile dressings soaked in a solution of **Hypericum** or **Hypercal** or **Urtica Urens**. The solution is made from 5ml (20 drops) of tincture in 200ml (half a pint) of cool, previously boiled, water.

Keep the dressing moist and disturb it as little as possible, renewing it every twelve hours or so, until the skin has healed. Apply **Calendula** ointment around the outside edge.

By Mouth

Shock and fear.	**Aconite 30c.** One dose every fifteen minutes for an hour. Repeat if necessary.
Pain: first degree with redness.	**Urtica Urens 6c.** One dose every fifteen minutes or when the pain returns. Stop with improvement.
Pain: second degree, with cracking skin and blistering.	**Causticum 6c.** One dose every two hours until relief.
Pain: third degree, with destruction of deeper tissues.	**Cantharis 6c.** One dose every two hours until relief.

EYE INJURIES – BLOWS TO THE EYE

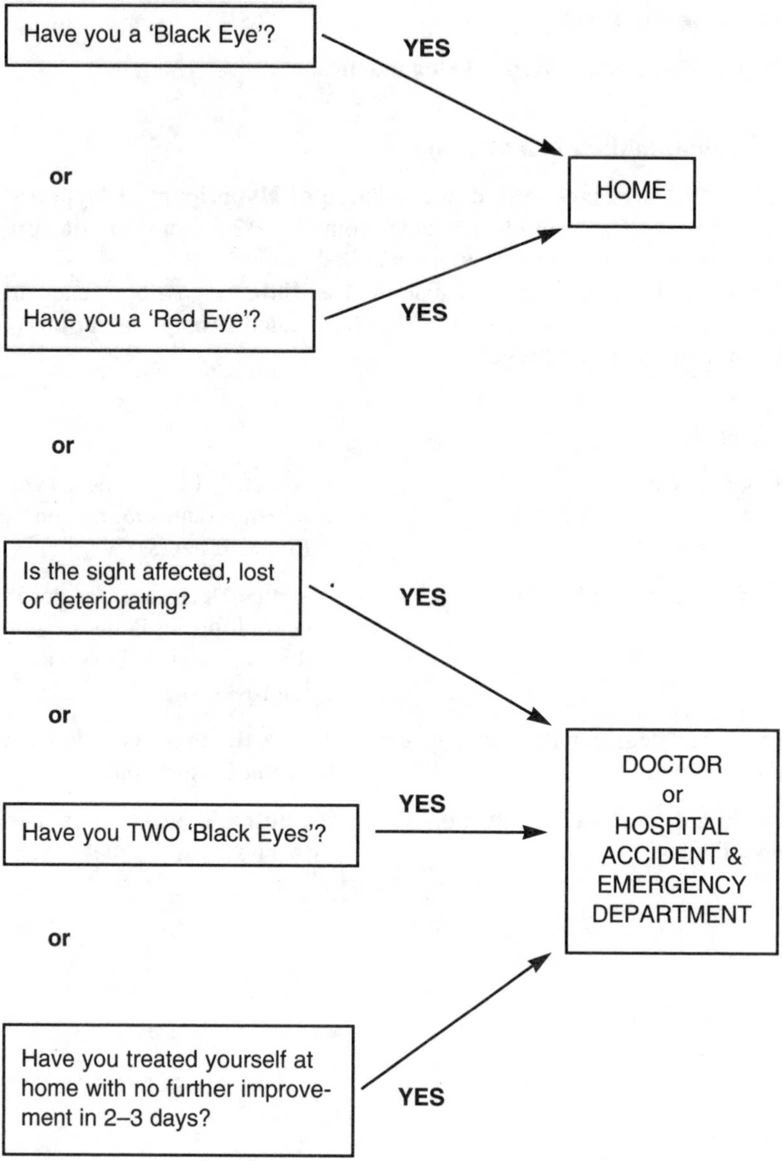
Have you a 'Black Eye'?
YES
HOME
or
Have you a 'Red Eye'?
YES
or
Is the sight affected, lost or deteriorating?
YES
or
Have you TWO 'Black Eyes'?
YES
DOCTOR or HOSPITAL ACCIDENT & EMERGENCY DEPARTMENT
or
Have you treated yourself at home with no further improvement in 2–3 days?
YES

EYE INJURIES – BLOWS TO THE EYE

Black Eye

Bruising around the eye margins with or without swelling.

Bruising (swelling) with pain.	**Arnica 6c.** One dose every two hours for 5–6 doses.
Bruising with pain. Better for cold applications.	**Ledum 6c.** One dose every two hours for 5–6 doses.
Pain in the eyeball.	**Symphytum 6c.** One dose every two hours for 5–6 doses.
Continuing pain and sensitivity externally.	**Hypericum 6c** or **Symphytum 6c.** One dose every two to three hours until the pain is reduced.

'Conjunctivitis'

Inflammation of the outer layer covering the white of the eye.	**Euphrasia tincture in a solution.** Bathe the eye with this solution which is made up of two drops of the tincture in an eye bath of cold (previously boiled) water.

'Red Eye'

A thin layer of bright red blood in the corner of the eye.	**Hamamelis 6c.** First day one dose every 2–3 hours. Later three times a day for 2–3 days.

EYE INJURIES – FOREIGN BODIES

Treat the eyes with great respect, and treat eye injuries very seriously.

Foreign Body in the Eye

Any particle, be it dust, stone, metal or whatever, must be removed, because of the possibility of infection and the loss of sight in that eye.

If hammering or using a power drill caused the accident, a minute particle of metal may have penetrated the eyeball.

If in doubt, visit your doctor or a hospital Accident & Emergency Department immediately.

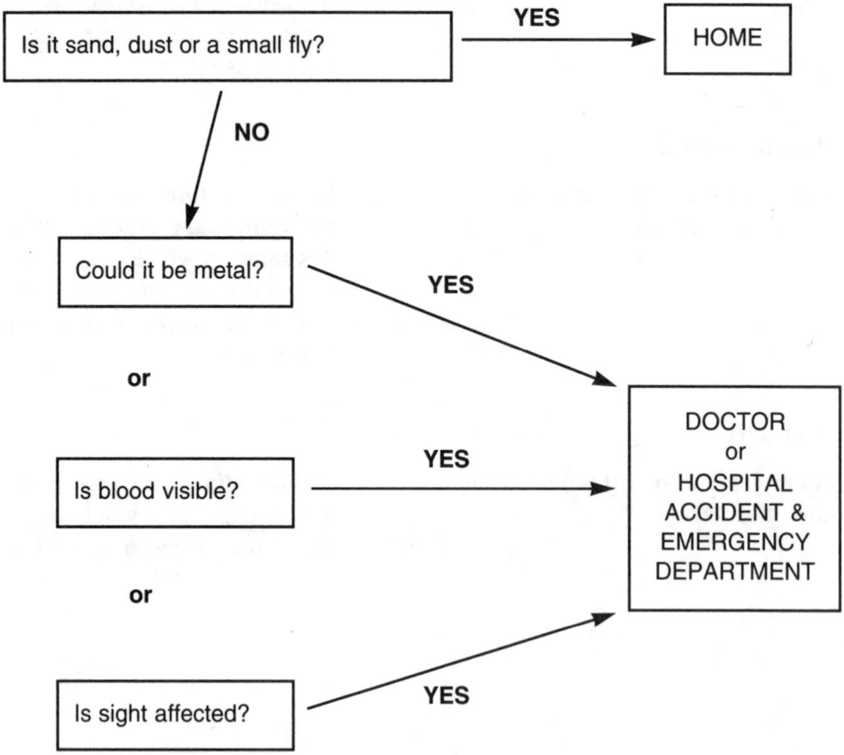

EYE INJURIES – FOREIGN BODIES

By Mouth

Shock and fear e.g. in a child.	**Aconite 30c.** One dose every half hour for 3–4 doses.
Pain and great sensitivity.	**Hypericum 6c.** One dose every half hour for 5–6 doses and as necessary afterwards.
Distress and 'hysterical' anxiety, e.g. in a child.	**Ignatia 30c** or **6c.** One dose every half hour for 3–4 doses.

Application to the Eye

Soreness may be relieved by:	**Euphrasia tincture in a solution**

Bathe the eye with this solution, which is made up of two drops of the eye drops in an eye bath of cold, previously boiled, water.

Remember, if the particle is firmly embedded, go to your doctor or to the Accident & Emergency Department, **without delay**.

FRACTURES

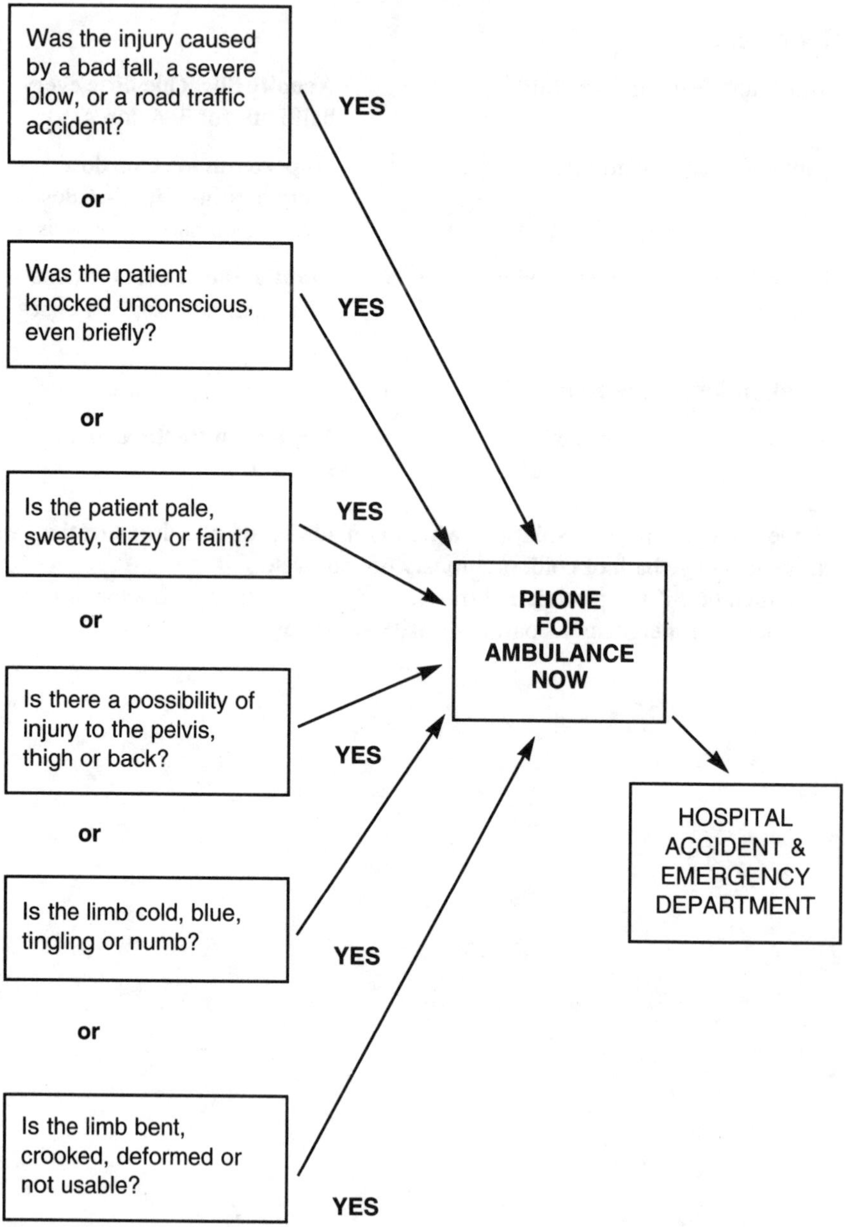
Was the injury caused by a bad fall, a severe blow, or a road traffic accident?
YES
or
Was the patient knocked unconscious, even briefly?
YES
or
Is the patient pale, sweaty, dizzy or faint?
YES
or
Is there a possibility of injury to the pelvis, thigh or back?
YES
or
Is the limb cold, blue, tingling or numb?
YES
or
Is the limb bent, crooked, deformed or not usable?
YES
PHONE FOR AMBULANCE NOW
HOSPITAL ACCIDENT & EMERGENCY DEPARTMENT

FRACTURES

Immediate First Aid

While arrangements are made to remove the casualty to hospital.

Shock. Nervous reaction. Physical reaction – pallor, cold sweat, dizziness, nausea.	**Aconite 30c.** One dose at once and 2–3 times more if needed.
Bruising – aching pain. Injury to muscles and soft tissues.	**Arnica 6c.** One dose after Aconite and then every half hour. You may give Arnica and Aconite alternately for 2 or 3 doses.

Home Treatment after Hospital Treatment

Bruising	**Arnica 6c.** One dose twice a day. Stop with improvement.
To strengthen the bones.	**Calcarea Phosphorica 6c.** One dose a day for 1–2 months.
Bone pain – along the bone or at the site of the break.	**Ruta 6c.** One dose twice a day for 2–3 weeks.
To speed healing.	**Symphytum 6c.** One dose twice a day for 2–3 weeks.

HEAD INJURY

Most people bang their heads at some time or another, and, beyond 'seeing stars' and suffering local tenderness and bruising, there are no other problems. So the *story* of the accident and the severity of the blow is most important in evaluating the situation.

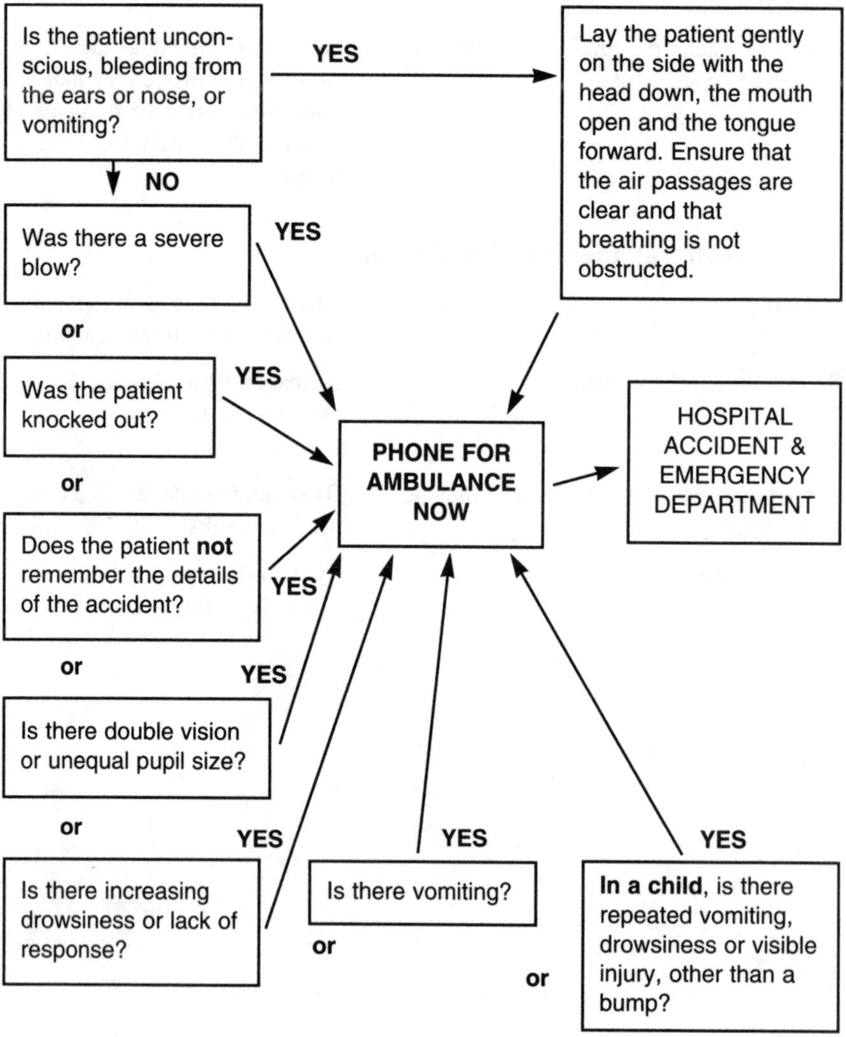

HEAD INJURY

Immediate First Aid

While the patient is being transported to the hospital A&E Department or arrangements are being made, you may give the following remedies:

Shock and fear.	**Aconite 30c.** One dose immediately and repeat if the symptoms return.
Bruising. Pain. Shock.	**Arnica 6c.** One dose every half hour for 5–6 doses.
Drowsiness. Lethargy. Lack of response. Unconsciousness.	**Opium 6c.** One dose every half hour until response.

Later Treatment

Remedies commonly given after any head injury.	**Arnica 6c** or **Natrum Sulphuricum 6c.** One dose twice a day for 5–7 days.
Continuing headaches.	**Natrum Sulphuricum 30c.** One dose two to three times a day for 5–7 days.

If any symptoms persist (or return) or if you are simply unhappy with the progress of the patient, consult your own doctor.

INSECT BITES AND STINGS

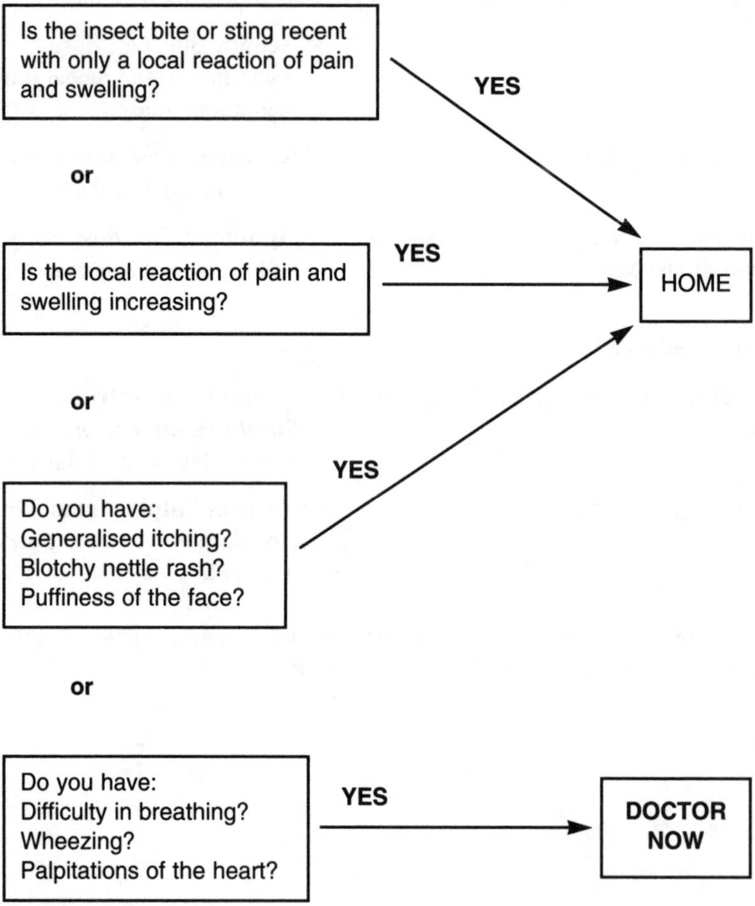

INSECT BITES AND STINGS

By Mouth

Shock and nervousness. Numbness and tingling. Hot, dry, burning skin.	**Aconite 30c.** One dose immediately and every half hour for 2–3 doses.
Particularly for wasp and bee stings, when hot, red and swollen.	**Apis 6c.** One dose every hour until improvement.
Irritation locally. Burning and stinging.	**Cantharis 6c.** One dose immediately and then every hour until soothed.
Chilly sensation, but better with *cold* applications, worse with warm applications. Worse for jarring or motion.	**Ledum 6c.** One dose every two hours for 3–5 doses.
Worse for cold, better with warmth. Irritable and sensitive to touch.	**Staphysagria 6c.** One dose every two hours until soothed.
Itchy, blotchy skin reaction; like nettle rash.	**Urtica Urens 6c.** One dose every hour until improvement.

Choose the most similar description and use that remedy. You may use two remedies alternately if you cannot make up your mind.

Application to the Bite or Sting

Bee, wasp, mosquito or midge bites and stings.	**Hypercal tincture.** Dab this on neat.

NOSEBLEEDS

Bleeding from the nose normally comes from a minor injury to the small veins in the lining of the soft part just inside the nostrils. Occasionally it occurs because of a virus infection – more frequently in children – and may start with sneezing.

Some people have a tendency to get nosebleeds easily, and while not serious, they are a nuisance. The following method of first aid is practical, and the most suitable remedy can be given at the beginning.

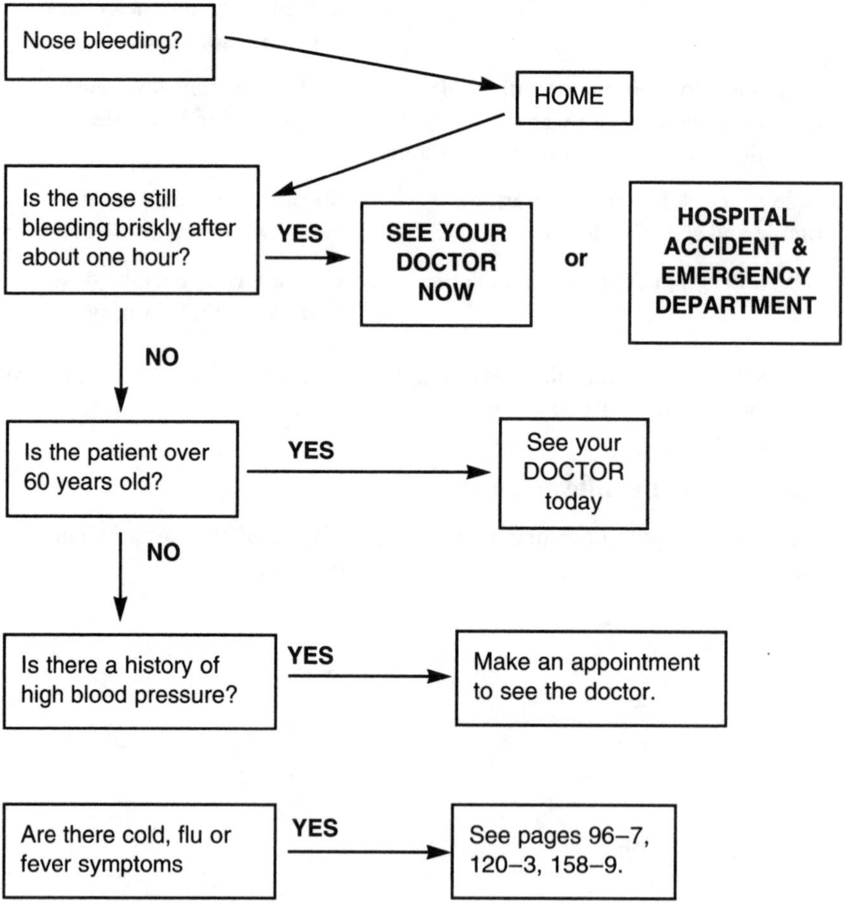

NOSEBLEEDS

General Measures

- *Do not panic. Be calm.* Give the remedy.
- Sit the patient down leaning forward, over a large bowl or basin, and tell him not to sniff or swallow the blood.
- Use a towel as a bib to cover the chest and drape it over the knees.
- Tell the patient to *pinch* the soft part of the nose between the thumb and forefinger for *not less than five minutes by the clock*, and to breathe through the mouth throughout.
- Do not blow the nose for *twelve* hours at least.

By Mouth

Irritable. Fear – 'something must be done'.	**Aconite 30c.** One dose every half hour for 2–3 doses.
After injury.	**Arnica 6c.** One dose every two to three hours for the first day and twice a day for 3 days.
Anxious, dithery and trembly, wants to be held.	**Gelsemium 6c.** One dose every half hour for 2–3 doses.
Weeping. 'Hysterical'.	**Ignatia 30c.** One dose every half hour for 2–3 doses.
Bright red bleeding, particularly after injury.	**Phosphorus 6c.** One dose every fifteen minutes until stopped.

SPRAINS AND STRAINS OF JOINTS, MUSCLES AND LIGAMENTS

Joints are movable only in certain directions and the ligaments and the tissues surrounding them are easily damaged if the joint is forced into an unusual position in an accident. The ligaments may then be stretched (strain), or partly torn (sprain), or completely torn. In extreme cases the bones may be fractured or dislocated.

In all cases, sprains and strains go together with pain and swelling of the joint. The swelling lasts up to three days or so but goes down over the next ten to fourteen days. Total healing may take up to two months or more if the injuries have been severe.

Use the remedies for injuries to muscle and ligaments also, since the treatment is essentially the same.

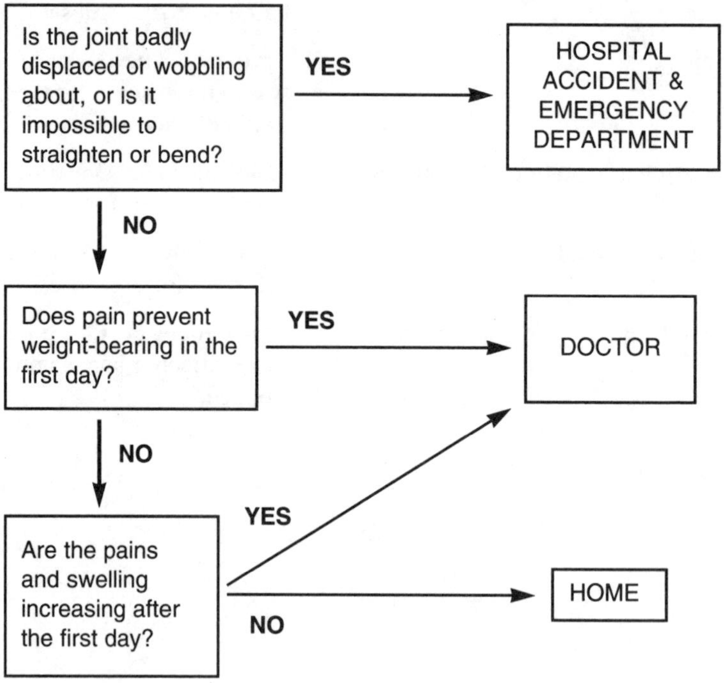

SPRAINS AND STRAINS OF JOINTS, MUSCLES AND LIGAMENTS

Immediate First Aid

While arrangements are being made to remove the casualty either to the hospital or the doctor:

- Stop all activity and weight bearing or strain.
- Reduce the swelling by applying an ice pack.
- Rest the joint in a comfortable, raised position.

By Mouth

Shock, fear or panic.	**Aconite 30c.** One dose every fifteen minutes for 3 doses.
Bruising and aching pain and shock.	**Arnica 6c.** One dose every fifteen minutes for 3 doses, then one every three or four hours a day for 3–4 days.

You may take Aconite and Arnica alternatively for the first three doses.

Swelling with the skin stretched tight. *Worse for touch and pressure.* Worse for heat.	**Apis 6c.** One dose every two to three hours on the first day, and then three times a day until improved.
Joint sprains	**Rhus Toxicodendron 6c.** Three times a day until swelling subsides.
Bruising of the bone. Better for warmth and movement of the joint. *Worse for cold and damp.*	**Ruta 6c.** One dose every two to three hours on the first day, and then three times a day until improved.

Application of Cream or Ointment to the Injury

Any of these creams or ointments can be rubbed or massaged into the skin over the injury.

Arnica. But not if the skin is broken.	**Ruta** or **Hamamelis** or **Rhus Toxicodendron.** These can be used if the skin is broken.

WOUNDS – ABRASIONS, SCRAPES AND GRAZES

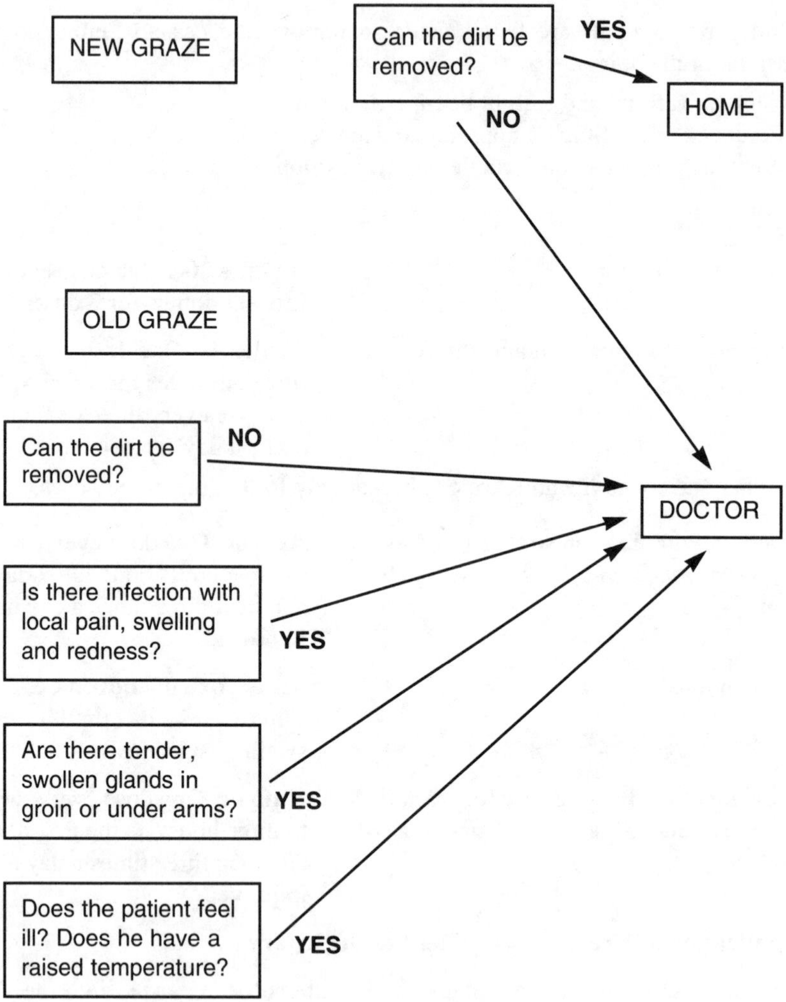

WOUNDS – ABRASIONS, SCRAPES AND GRAZES

Immediate First Aid

Wash the whole area in warm, soapy water, gently scrubbing grit and dirt out with a soft brush. Rinse under the cold water tap.

Apply a dressing soaked in **Calendula** lotion. This is made by adding 5ml (twenty drops) of tincture to 200ml (half a pint) of cool, previously boiled, water.

Application to the Wound

Keep the dressing moist with the same solution (freshly made).

After two or three changes of dressings in the first day or so, disturb the dressings as little as possible. One change a day will usually be adequate.

Later, **Calendula** ointment may be applied when the scab has formed.

By Mouth

For possible infection and to stimulate the healing process.	**Calendula 6c.** One dose immediately and then four times a day for 3–5 days.
If the graze is sensitive, painful, involving areas rich in nerves (e.g. finger ends).	**Hypericum 6c.** One dose three times a day for 2–3 days.
Later, if there is infection with yellow pus.	**Hepar Sulphuris 6c.** One dose three times a day for 3–4 days until clean.

WOUNDS – CUTS AND LACERATIONS

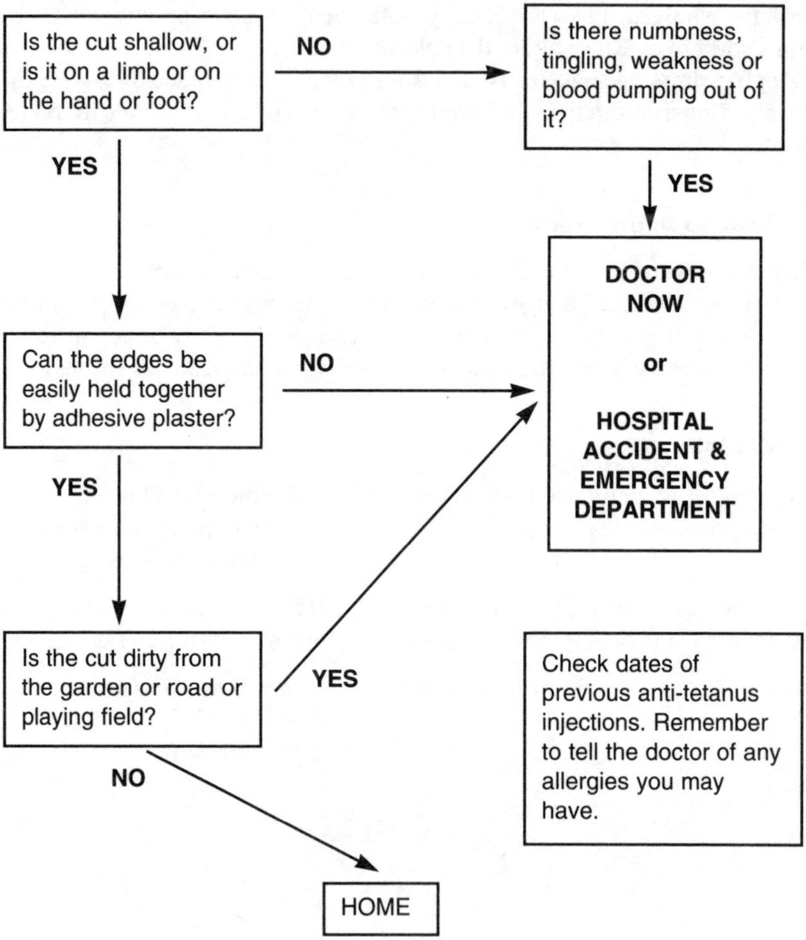
Is the cut shallow, or is it on a limb or on the hand or foot?
NO
Is there numbness, tingling, weakness or blood pumping out of it?
YES
YES
DOCTOR NOW
or
HOSPITAL ACCIDENT & EMERGENCY DEPARTMENT
Can the edges be easily held together by adhesive plaster?
NO
YES
Is the cut dirty from the garden or road or playing field?
YES
NO
HOME
Check dates of previous anti-tetanus injections. Remember to tell the doctor of any allergies you may have.

WOUNDS – CUTS AND LACERATIONS

Immediate First Aid

Wash the wound with warm, soapy water. If dirt is present, lightly scrub out the wound with a soft nail brush. Rinse under the cold tap.

Application to the Wound

Wash the cut with the freshly prepared **Calendula** or **Hypercal solution**. This is made by adding 5ml (20 drops) of the tincture of Calendula or Hypercal to 200ml (half a pint) of cool, previously boiled, water.

Dress the wound with a sterile, unmedicated dressing kept moistened with the Calendula or Hypercal solution. Change the dressing if it becomes soaked with blood, but later changing it once a day will be adequate. If the dressing sticks to the cut, soak it off with the prepared solution.

By Mouth

Shock.	**Aconite 30c.** One dose immediately and then three further doses at fifteen-minute intervals.
Bruising. Shock.	**Arnica 6c.** One dose after the Aconite, then two or three times a day for 2–3 days.
Bleeding. Possible infection. To promote healing.	**Calendula 6c.** One dose three times a day for 4–5 days.
Pain – especially parts normally very sensitive like fingers and lips.	**Hypericum 6c.** One dose three times a day until relief.

WOUNDS – INFECTED

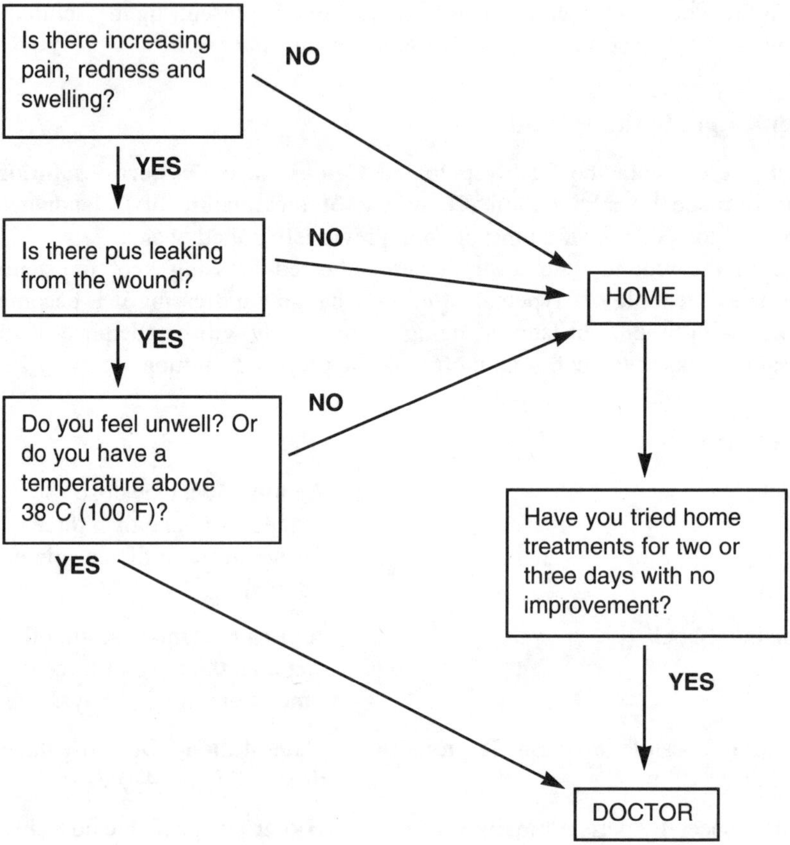

Remember to tell the doctor of any allergies you may have.

WOUNDS – INFECTED

Immediate First Aid

Wash out the wound using small pieces of sterile gauze or clean cotton material and a freshly made solution of **Calendula** or **Hypercal**. This is made by adding 5ml (20 drops) of the tincture of either of the above to 200ml (half a pint) of cool, previously boiled water.

Application to the Wound

Sterile dressings should be applied and kept moist with a fresh solution of either the Calendula or Hypercal. Later, **Calendula ointment** may be applied. Change the dressings two or three times a day to begin with. Change them less often as the pus gets less and the wound becomes cleaner.

By Mouth

Wound torn and jagged, with bruising and a bruised feeling.	**Arnica 6c.** One dose three to four times a day for 3–4 days.
To resist infection and to promote healing.	**Calendula 6c.** One dose immediately and three times a day for 3–4 days.
Infected wounds, yellow pus.	**Hepar Sulphuris 6c.** One dose three to four times a day till clean.
Pain and sensitivity.	**Hypericum 6c.** One dose three to four times a day for 2–3 days.

WOUNDS – PUNCTURED

Most puncture wounds are harmless, but occasionally dirt is introduced and causes deep infection. Sometimes pieces of a sharp object may be broken off, and X-rays may be needed to locate them. In cases of infection, antibiotics be required. Ensure that the person has had a tetanus injection **within the last ten years**.

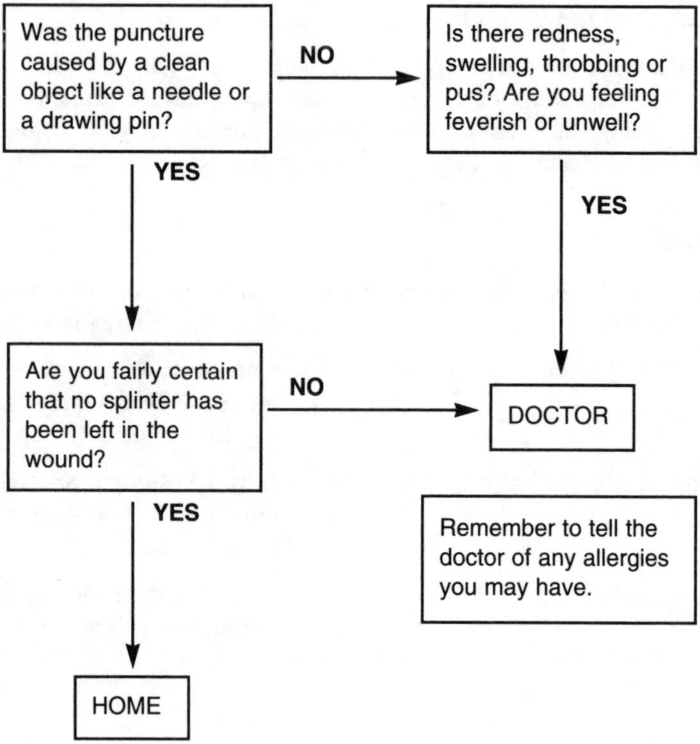

WOUNDS – PUNCTURED

Application to the Wound

Clean the wound and apply tincture of **Calendula** or tincture of **Hypercal**.

By Mouth

The basic remedy for puncture wounds is:	**Ledum 6c.** One dose immediately and three times a day for 3 days.
If the wound becomes infected, i.e. throbbing pain, redness, swelling or tenderness.	**Hepar Sulphuris 6c.** One dose three times a day until improvement, *or* **Ledum 6c.** One dose three times a day until improvement.
If a splinter remains in the wound:	**Silica 6c.** One dose four times a day until extruded.

If in any doubt, consult your doctor. He may decide that tetanus toxoid injections or antibiotics are needed. Continue to use the homoeopathic remedies as well.

– NOTES –

PROBLEMS OF WOMEN

Menstruation

Menstruation is the episode of bleeding which occurs about every month during the thirty or so years a woman is capable of becoming pregnant. It starts in adolescence (pages 40–1) and ends at the menopause (pages 64–6). The loss itself consists of blood and the broken-down lining of the womb, which is shed for three to five days.

A woman may have the same menstrual pattern for years, or it may be very variable. After a pregnancy there may be a new pattern which may be permanent or temporary. The pattern may also change because of illness, physical and mental stress, or for no obvious reason.

If the pattern changes, even for no obvious reason, do not be alarmed but wait for two or three cycles to pass. Very often the cycle reverts of its own accord to the old pattern and all is well. If the old pattern is not resumed, you must consult your doctor for investigation to exclude more serious problems.

From the start of periods in adolescence most women are affected by the rhythmical rise and fall of the hormones during the menstrual cycle. Although some hardly notice anything unusual, others may complain of mental and physical symptoms. Each woman responds to these hormonal changes in her own way. Irritability, tiredness, headache, depression and pain can occur before, during and after the bleeding in any combination.

Water retention will show itself in weight gain, and more particularly, as puffiness of the face, bloating, swelling and discomfort in the abdomen and swelling and tenderness of the breasts. (See 'Premenstrual Tension', pages 50–1 and 'Breast Problems', pages 52–3.)

Pain may be located in the womb, in the lower part of the abdomen, deep down in the pelvis, in the lower back, or down the thighs. (See 'Painful Periods', pages 44–5.)

When a woman has period problems, she must become accurate in recording the sequence of events each menstrual cycle over three or four months, so that a typical pattern can be recognised.

The *first day* of the last menstrual bleed counts as the *first day* of the new menstrual cycle.

The following list of symptoms and when they start and finish will be found to be helpful in choosing a remedy:

- Length of the cycle (number of days from the *first day* of the last menstrual bleed to the *first day* of the new menstrual cycle.
- Length of bleeding (number of days).
- Type of bleeding – e.g. heavy, light, red, black, clots.
- Type, time and place of pains.
- Headache – especially the time in relation to the bleeding.
- Feelings – depression, weepiness, irritability, anger, tiredness.
- Weight gain – swelling of stomach, breasts, hands and feet, and the face.
- Unusual symptoms. These may be of use to an experienced homoeopath in choosing a remedy if your own choice is not helpful.

Frequently the most effective time to take the remedies is on day twelve of the cycle, although some women may find that the day after the bleeding stops is easier to remember. If the last menstrual bleed was a long time before, and there is no question of the patient being pregnant, take the remedies immediately.

One of the remedies on the right-hand page of each section may be helpful, but the picture may be complicated by emotional problems and other factors. In this case, consult other relevant pages in this section of the book and try to form a composite picture. If this fails, seek the advice of a doctor, because careful medical examination and investigation may be necessary. If these are all clear, consult an experienced homoeopath for a wider-ranging homoeopathic evaluation.

ESTABLISHMENT OF MENSTRUAL PERIODS IN ADOLESCENT GIRLS

In Western society the age of the onset of menstruation is dropping steadily, so that even nine to ten years is increasingly common. If regular menstruation has not occurred by the middle teens, girls and their mothers become anxious. In other girls menstruation may have started normally, but later on becomes irregular, again giving rise to anxiety.

It is at this stage that the use of homoeopathic remedies is justified. However, a doctor should be consulted if their use is not successful within a few months, because he may have to examine the girl to see whether causes other than those amenable to homoeopathy may be present.

If it is possible that the patient is pregnant the question of restarting the periods does not arise. The pregnancy should be confirmed by your own doctor and ante-natal care started.

HEAVY PERIODS – FLOODING (MENORRHAGIA)

Heavy bleeding may or may not be painful. The fact that there is no pain *does not* mean that the underlying cause may not be serious. Tumours, fibroids, polyps, early miscarriage and hormonal imbalance must be thought of.

If heavy bleeding occurs on more than one occasion, the patient must consult her doctor. The doctor may decide that blood and smear tests would be helpful, and after an evaluation of the results in the light of the history, that a gynaecologist should be consulted.

While the patient waits for all this to happen, or when serious disease has been excluded, the use of homoeopathic remedies can very often modify or completely control the situation. The choice of the remedy should be based on the type of bleeding, the character of the pain, if present, and the more general characteristics of the patient.

ESTABLISHMENT OF MENSTRUAL PERIODS IN ADOLESCENT GIRLS

Mild, gentle, timid. Pains, moods, mind changeable. Weeps easily, loves sympathy. Seeks attention. Jealous. Generally feels better in fresh air and for gentle exercise.	**Pulsatilla 30c.** Three doses, one morning, evening and the following morning, starting on day twelve of the cycle.
Irregular, variable bleeding. Premenstrual bloating. Moodiness, depression, irritability. Generally better for vigorous exercise.	**Sepia 30c.** Three doses, one morning, evening and the following morning, starting on day twelve of the cycle.

HEAVY PERIODS – FLOODING (MENORRHAGIA)

Hot, bright red blood loss. Painful cramps.	**Belladonna 6c.** One dose three times a day while still bleeding.
Bright red bleeding on least exertion. Previous periods normal. Face and lips pale, flushing on exertion.	**Ferrum Metallicum 6c.** One dose three times a day during the period while still bleeding.
Heavy loss of bright red blood and clots. Changed character of bleeding, also bright red bleeding between periods. Nausea.	**Ipecacuanha 6c.** One dose three times a day while still bleeding.
Heavy bleeding, often late. Bearing down pains, eased by crossing legs. Low backache eased by movement.	**Sepia 6c.** One dose three times a day while still bleeding.

The remedies for this condition may also be given as three doses, one morning, evening and the following morning, starting on day twelve of the menstrual cycle. In this case, use the 30c potency. Observe the effects over three menstrual cycles, and consult your doctor if the symptoms have not cleared up by then.

LATE PERIODS

Some women have a natural menstrual cycle which is longer than the average of twenty-eight days. This is normal for them and should not cause concern, provided that they remain well and happy.

However, some women develop delayed periods and this may make them unwell. These periods may be painful and abnormal, as a result of hormonal imbalance. This itself may arise from emotional causes, the use of the contraceptive pill, or the onset of the menopause.

Premenstrual tension occurs or increases sometimes, and this is dealt with separately (see pages 50–1).

One of the remedies on the opposite page may be helpful, but the picture may be complicated by emotional problems, different types of pain, and feelings of malaise before, during or after the bleeding. If this is so, consult the other relevant pages in this section of the book and try to form a composite picture. If this fails, seek the advice of an experienced homoeopath.

LATE PERIODS

Late – after fright or chilling, (especially in young girls whose periods are not properly established).	**Aconite 30c**
Blood pale. Painful colic. Generally unwell and constipated. 'Morning sickness' during period.	**Graphites 6c**
Black, tarry blood. Flows lying down and stops flowing on walking about. Heartburn and belching.	**Magnesium Carbonicum 30c**
Suppressed due to shock or grief.	**Natrum Muriaticum 30c**
Thick, dark and clotted. Intermittent flow. Painful pressure downwards. Gentle, yielding; highly emotional; loves sympathy; weepy, changeable; easily discouraged; feels better in open air.	**Pulsatilla 30c**
Hot, flushing skin, rashes and spots. Faint feeling in late morning.	**Sulphur 6c**

Dosage. All the remedies for this condition may best be given as three doses, one morning, evening and the following morning, starting on day twelve of the menstrual cycle.

PAINFUL PERIODS (DYSMENORRHOEA)

The pain may be located in the womb, low down within the pelvis, higher in the abdomen, or in the low back. It may spread to the thighs.

One of the remedies on the opposite page may be helpful, but the picture may be complicated by emotional problems, different types of pain, and feelings of malaise before, during or after the bleeding. If this is so, consult the other relevant pages in this section of the book and try to form a composite picture. If this fails, seek the advice of an experienced homoeopath.

PAINFUL PERIODS (DYSMENORRHOEA)

Severe pain – sudden onset. Nervous restlessness.	**Aconite 30c.** One dose, at fifteen to thirty minute intervals. Stop with improvement.
Cutting pain the day before period starts. Pressing down pain in right pelvis. Hot, profuse bright red bleeding. Usually better moving about.	**Belladonna 6c.** One dose, at fifteen to thirty minute intervals. Stop with improvement.
Spasms of severe pain in the womb on the first day of bleeding; may seem to spread to other parts of the body. Light bleeding.	**Caulophyllum 6c.** One dose, at fifteen to thirty minute intervals. Stop with improvement.
Labour-like pains. Blood brown with clots. Peevish, impatient, irritable. 'Can't bear it.' 'Not fair.'	**Chamomilla 6c.** One dose, at fifteen to thirty minute intervals. Stop with improvement.
Spasms of colic, relieved by hot water bottle. Dark, stringy blood.	**Magnesium Phosphoricum 6c.** One dose, at fifteen to thirty minute intervals. Stop with improvement.
Cutting, tearing pains in lower abdomen and back. Chilly sensation. Diarrhoea during period. Tearful.	**Pulsatilla 6c.** One dose, at fifteen to thirty minute intervals. Stop with improvement.
Dragging down pain in left side of pelvis. Downwards pressure. Must cross legs. Bleeding early or late, scanty or profuse.	**Sepia 6c.** One dose, at fifteen to thirty minute intervals. Stop with improvement.

The remedies for this condition may also be given as three doses, one morning, evening and the following morning, starting on day twelve of the menstrual cycle. Use the 30c potency.

SCANTY PERIODS

(A regular cycle, but the flow is short-lasting and small in quantity.)

Generally, scanty periods are not a sign of ill-health. If the patient remains well and happy, then do nothing. If she feels unwell in any way, the use of a homoeopathic remedy may help.

One of the remedies on the page opposite may be helpful, but the picture may be complicated by emotional problems, different types of pain, and feelings of malaise before, during or after the bleeding. If this is so, consult the other relevant pages in this section of the book and try to form a composite picture. If this fails, seek the advice of a homoeopath.

SCANTY PERIODS

Caused by sudden chill or shock.	**Aconite 30c**
Pale and chilly, fat and flabby.	**Calcarea Carbonica 30c**
Nervous, 'uptight'; holds emotions in; depression, lack of confidence. Periods may also be irregular and never established properly.	**Natrum Muriaticum 30c**
Pale, thin, vivacious, but nervous and fearful. Demands constant reassurance.	**Phosphorus 30c**
Weak, pale, gentle; moody and tearful; easily discouraged.	**Pulsatilla 30c**
Low abdominal, or bearing down pain. Possibly constipated. Irritable, depressed; wants to be alone.	**Sepia 30c**

Dosage: All the remedies for this condition may best be given as three doses, morning, evening and the following morning, starting on day twelve of the menstrual cycle.

PREMENSTRUAL SYNDROME (PMS)
PREMENSTRUAL TENSION (PMT)

Most women can recognise when a period is about to start. Some women find that for several days before a period they become unwell. These are the more common problems which occur:

- Emotional changes: irritability, depression, frustration, jealousy, 'nastiness', loss of affection for family, weeping easily for no reason.
- Fluid retention: weight gain, bloated stomach, swollen breasts, swollen hands.
- Pain: womb, deep inside pelvis, low back, thighs, headache, breasts.

In recent years women have been helped by hormone therapy, diuretics (drugs to remove retained water) and Vitamin B_6. Some women have found that Oil of Evening Primrose has been of help.

Only homoeopathic treatment, however, can actually cure the whole distressing syndrome by apparently re-establishing the correct hormone balance. Sometimes this is done within one or two menstrual cycles, and sometimes after several cycles. The patterns of symptoms to the left on the page opposite relate to four of the most commonly needed homoeopathic remedies in these situations. Their names are on the right.

Use the remedy in a 30c potency, giving one dose morning and evening and the next morning, starting on day twelve of the cycle, or at the end of a period. Use only three doses each month.

You may get a good response by finding that the expected unpleasant symptoms do not occur, or are reduced in severity. Occasionally, some symptoms (e.g. headache) may be shifted from before the period to after it. Do not be alarmed by this, but continue the treatment month by month until the symptoms have been cleared.

Then stop the remedy.

After a few symptom-free or relatively symptom-free cycles, the problems may partly return. When this occurs, *repeat the three doses for one cycle only, and wait.*

Usually the improvement tends to last for greater lengths of time and eventually only a very occasional use of the remedy is needed. Sometimes a patient may need to take the remedy in alternate cycles, or every third cycle.

If you are not able to get relief, consult an experienced homoeopath.

PREMENSTRUAL SYNDROME (PMS)
PREMENSTRUAL TENSION (PMT)

Hands swollen. Clumsy and drops things. Clothes tight, needs to loosen them. Hates tight things around the neck. Spiteful, vindictive, jealous. Unreasonable. Deliberately nasty and desires to hurt; hates herself afterwards. Talkative. Better after bleeding starts and may pass a lot of urine then. Worse in the morning or on waking from a nap.	**Lachesis 30c**
Bloated stomach. Swollen, tender breasts. Low abdominal pain. Moody. Negative, irritable. Selfish. Dissatisfied. Self-pitying. Blames others. Pessimistic. Takes it out on family. Hates sympathy but demands it.	**Natrum Muriaticum 30c**
Swollen breasts. Irregular periods. Thick white vaginal discharge before periods. Changeable and contradictory. Tearful. Peevish. Jealous. Loves sympathy. Over-sensitive and easily hurt. Better after gentle exercise in fresh air. Worse in stuffy atmosphere.	**Pulsatilla 30c**
Breasts swollen, tender. Bearing down sensation eased by crossing legs. Womb feels as if falling out. Irregular periods. Weary, droopy, overwhelmed. Dislikes family and partner – doesn't want them. Loss of libido. Worse mid-afternoon. Better after vigorous exercise or dancing.	**Sepia 30c**

Dosage: Read the discussion on the opposite page carefully.

Vaginal Discharge (Leucorrhoea)

A slight discharge from the vagina is normally present in most women, and is white to pale yellow in colour. However, if it is excessive, offensive in smell, soils the underwear excessively, or is irritating or bloodstained, medical advice must be taken.

The discharge is often, but not always, due to an infection. If there is any reason to think that it may have been caught from sexual intercourse, then the patient and the sexual partner should go to the Genito-Urinary Medicine (GUM) Department at a local hospital as soon as possible, because of the specialised laboratory facilities they have. It is not necessary to book an appointment or have a letter of referral.

In some cases medical treatment may not help, or only be helpful for a short time.

Provided that serious disease has been excluded by the appropriate medical specialists, homoeopathic medicine may be more beneficial than orthodox medical treatments.

The remedies and dosage scheme on the page opposite will be helpful in the short term. It must be stressed, however, that for permanent benefit the patient should consult a homoeopath, who will treat the problem 'constitutionally'. Discharges of this nature often have an underlying constitutional origin, which the homoeopath is able to treat holistically, with every expectation of cure. A longstanding problem such as this may well take a long time to resolve.

Attention to hygiene and to general health is important. Avoid the use of strong antiseptics, soaps and deodorants, as sensitivity reactions may occur. Ask for 'Simple Soap' at your chemist and wash with it.

A solution of **Calendula** can be made up by adding 5ml (20 drops) of the tincture of Calendula to 200ml (half a pint) of cool, previously boiled water, and bathing with it.

VAGINAL DISCHARGE (LEUCORRHOEA)

Thrush. Continuous minor discomfort or recurring bouts of reinfection. Profuse, thick, creamy discharge. Severe itching and soreness.	**Helonias 6c**
Yellow, thick, ropey, sticky. Soreness, rawness, itching.	**Hydrastis 6c**
Smelly, yellow, staining. Burning pain, rawness, violent itching.	**Kreosotum 6c**
Greenish, slimy. Burning and itching. Burning urge to urinate.	**Mercurius Solubilis 6c**
Smelly, brownish-yellow discharge. Itching, pricking pain in ulcers.	**Nitric Acid 6c**
Bland discharge or thick, yellowy-green; usually non-irritant but can be irritant sometimes.	**Pulsatilla 6c**
Jelly, white or yellow. Burning pain. Or dryness with discomfort when walking.	**Sepia 6c**

Dosage: All the remedies for this condition may best be given as one dose morning and evening, reducing with improvement. Stop when the discharge clears. If there is no improvement, consult a homoeopath.

Breast Problems

BREAST PAIN

Breast pain is a common problem in the pre-menstrual phase of the cycle. As long as the pain completely resolves after the menstrual period, it can be safely treated homoeopathically. If the pain persists the doctor must be consulted.

All women should learn to examine their own breasts regularly so that they will be in a position to detect any changes and seek medical advice. Self-examination can be taught by the Practice Nurse, and leaflets are available from your surgery.

LUMPY BREASTS (NODULES)

As with breast pain, breasts often become lumpy in the premenstrual phase. As long as the lumps completely resolve *after* the menstrual period, this condition can be safely treated homoeopathically. However, if in any doubt, **seek medical advice**.

BREAST PAIN

Breasts tend to be hard and tender. Stitching pain in nipples. Better for pressure. After a blow or fall on the breast. (Use Arnica first.)	**Conium 6c** or **30c.** One dose 3–4 times a day. Reduce with improvement.
Breasts hard and sensitive. Better for warmth. Worse for damp and motion.	**Phytolacca 6c** or **30c.** One dose 3–4 times a day. Reduce with improvement.

LUMPY BREASTS (NODULES)

Throbbing pain in heavy breast. Lumps in breast – pain worse lying down. Worse with touch or jarring.	**Belladonna 6c.** One dose 4–5 times a day. Reduce with improvement.
Darting pains in breast. Tender lumps.	**Carbo Animalis 6c.** One dose 4–5 times a day. Reduce with improvement.
Breasts painful to touch, either shrunken or enlarged, worse before and during periods. Stitching pain in nipples. Worse lying down. Better for pressure and motion.	**Conium 6c.** One dose 4–5 times a day. Reduce with improvement.
Breasts hard, painful and purple coloured. Very sensitive to touch. Lumps in breast, with or without swollen glands in armpits.	**Phytolacca 6c.** One dose 4–5 times a day. Reduce with improvement.

Pregnancy

For this section the arrangement of left- and right-hand pages has not been followed. Problems which may occur in pregnancy are listed with possible remedies.

Homoeopathic treatment will help greatly, but it must not in any way be regarded as a substitute for the usual ante-natal and post-natal care provided by your general practitioner and midwife.

THREATENED MISCARRIAGE

Causes Known or Suspected

Miscarriage may be caused by hormone imbalance or a fall, heavy lifting or the general overexertion and tiredness of a mother with a young family. Situations like this can threaten to destroy a pregnancy. So, particularly in women with a previous history of miscarriage or threatened miscarriage, these situations should be avoided or prevented.

The signs of a threatened miscarriage are bleeding and painful contractions. When the condition seems to develop:

- Go to bed,
- Rest,
- Take the appropriate remedy, and
- **Call the doctor**.

Hormone imbalance is frequently the cause of recurring miscarriage, especially in the early weeks of pregnancy. In this situation the patient must be cared for by an obstetrician. 'A show' or 'spotting' refers to the loss of a small amount of blood, perhaps only sufficient to soil underwear.

A *fall*, followed by aching or pain in the womb with bleeding – 'a show', or 'spotting', perhaps mucus, or a loss of clear fluid.	**Arnica 6c**, or **Arnica 30c** if it is available.
Heavy lifting, resulting in dragging pain with restlessness, pressure and tenderness in pelvis, bleeding – 'a show'.	**Cinnamon 6c**
Overexertion with family commitments, generally weary and tired, backache, restlessness.	**Rhus Toxicodendron 6c**

Shock

Great shock and terror; wakes with nightmares; contractions start; show of blood.	**Aconite 30c**
Nervous, emotional; acute hysterical reaction; weeping; extremely restless; irregular uterine pain.	**Ignatia 30c**
Nervous emotional prostration; overcome by depression.	**Opium 6c**

Dosage: All remedies should be one dose *every hour* until improvement, and then three times a day for 3–4 days.

MORNING SICKNESS

Nausea with faintness and vomiting, yawning. Dislike of food, drink and smell of tobacco smoke and food. Worse after loss of sleep or emotional disturbances or travelling.	**Cocculus 6c** or **30c.** One dose every 2–4 hours. Reduce with improvement.
Persistent nausea, great salivation; vomiting with no thirst and clean tongue. Vomiting does not relieve nausea. Irritable and peevish. Worse warmth of room. Better open air and rest.	**Ipecacuanha 6c** or **30c.** One dose every 2–4 hours. Reduce with improvement.
Constipation. Retching with belching and nausea marked. Very little vomiting, but if so usually immediately after eating. Nausea all day long with no vomiting. Chilly and irritable.	**Nux Vomica 6c** or **30c.** One dose every 2–4 hours. Reduce with improvement.
Great nausea with smell of food. Nausea before eating in morning. Empty sensation in stomach, better by eating. Exhausted, apathetic personality, drooping physically. Sallow and pallid. Likes acid flavours. Dislikes milk and the smell of cooking. Better for exercise and dancing.	**Sepia 6c** or **30c.** One dose every 2–4 hours. Reduce with improvement.

HEARTBURN

Acidity with sour taste in mouth, with sour belching. Dislikes milk, boiled foods and fat. Likes raw, indigestible foods, eggs and sweets. Worse while eating.	**Calcarea Carbonica 6c** or **30c.** One dose every 1–2 hours. Stop with improvement.
Acid burning, great flatulence with water brash. Much thirst but drinking causes shuddering. Craving for stimulants. Vomiting.	**Capsicum 6c** or **30c.** One dose every 1–2 hours. Stop with improvement.
Very irritable and angry. Sour belching. Nausea after foods. Feels like a weight in stomach. Bloated feelings. Generally worse after coffee.	**Nux Vomica 6c** or **30c.** One dose every 1–2 hours. Stop with improvement.
Heartburn with nausea. Worse after warm, rich, fatty foods and drinks. Not thirsty. Food tastes salty but has bitter taste in mouth. Vomits food eaten long before. Prefers cold foods and drinks, but may vomit ice cream.	**Pulsatilla 6c** or **30c.** One dose every 1–2 hours. Stop with improvement.

CRAVINGS

Note: Cravings in pregnancy are usual. Only use the following remedies if your cravings are becoming a problem to you.

Salty foods, extra salt. Patient has flatulence and belching.	**Carbo Vegetabilis 6c**
Wants a variety of indigestible things; craves sour things. Moods changeable.	**Ignatia 6c**
Sweets, sugar, sweet foods, chocolate. Patient has rumbling wind.	**Lycopodium 6c**
Pickles, sour foods and drinks; vinegar.	**Sepia 6c**
Sweets, sugar, sweet foods, fat and butter.	**Sulphur 6c**

Dosage: One dose at intervals of one to two hours, as long as is necessary.

NIGHT CRAMPS

Intolerable cramping with numbness and muscular twitching. Worse between 9 p.m. and midnight. Temperamental, over-sensitive to pain, angry and rude. Worse with anger and lying in bed.	**Chamomilla 6c**
Agitation and shooting pains like electric shocks with muscular soreness and stiffness. Better from local warmth. Restless feeling with heavy aching and muscular soreness in limbs.	**Cimicifuga 6c**
Overactive mind; unable to sleep; restlessness. Severe cramps. Better for pressure. Worse for movement and at night.	**Coffea Cruda 6c**
Violent cramps and spasms (especially in calves and feet) start and end suddenly. Worse at night, and by movement and touch. Weary feeling in legs.	**Cuprum Metallicum 6c**
Legs numb and feel paralysed and stiff. Cramp in calves and soles. Shooting pain from toes to thighs.	**Nux Vomica 6c**

Dosage: One dose before retiring to bed. Repeat nightly. Stop with improvement.

URINARY FREQUENCY

See also 'Cystitis', pages 128–9.

Constant urging to pass urine. Burning and scalding pain before, during, and after passing urine. Persistent griping pain in bladder and dribbling.	**Cantharis 6c** or **30c.** One dose every 1–2 hours. Reduce with improvement.
Leaking of urine with coughing, lifting or exertion or when asleep. Unable to pass urine normally and regularly; i.e. retention of urine after labour.	**Causticum 6c** or **30c.** One dose every 3–4 times a day. Reduce with improvement.
Urination leading to burning pain. Sensation of incomplete emptying of bladder. Usually a catheter has been used during confinement, but may be due to stretching during delivery.	**Staphysagria 6c** or **30c.** One dose 3 or 4 times a day. Reduce with improvement.

BACKACHE

Bruised feeling. Difficulty in walking. From overexertion.	**Arnica 6c** or **30c.** One dose two or three times a day.
Weakness and dragging feeling in small of the back. (Can also be used after the confinement.)	**Kali Carbonicum 6c.** One dose two or three times a day for two or three days. Stop with improvement.
Marked weakness with not too much pain.	**Phosphoric Acid 6c.** One dose two or three times a day.
Very stiff, especially after rest. Improves with continued movement.	**Rhus Toxicodendron 6c.** One or two doses on each occasion.

EMOTIONAL DISTURBANCES – before and after confinement

'Cravings'. Craves unusual foods and is better for having them. Rapid changes of mood; contrary. Sensation of a lump in the throat. Constant sighing.	**Ignatia 30c.** One dose, at intervals of two to four hours, for 2–4 doses, and then three to four times a day for 2–3 days.
Indifference but loves sympathy. Feels better for being massaged. Afraid of being alone, the dark, thunder. Wants iced drinks, loves salt.	**Phosphorus 30c.** One dose once or twice a day for 2 or 3 days.
Moody, changeable; shy and tearful; loves sympathy. Dislikes fat, meat, butter, milk. Wants sour refreshing drinks. Better for fresh air and for gentle exercise.	**Pulsatilla 30c.** One dose 2–3 times a day for 2 or 3 days.
Indifferent to husband and children, loses interest. Depressed; bursts into tears with sympathy; 'want to get away'. Morning sickness; nausea with smell of cooking; loves chocolate, sour drinks and vinegar. Better for dancing and exercise.	**Sepia 30c.** One dose 3–4 times a day for 2 or 3 days.

COMING UP TO CONFINEMENT – from eight months (36 weeks)

To Calm False Labour Pains

Sharp pains across the abdomen.	**Cimicifuga 6c.** One dose at intervals of 30 minutes to one hour for 2–4 doses. Repeat if necessary.

To Allay Anxiety and Fear

Anxiety tending to fear or panic. Fear of death in confinement. Palpitations. Pins and needles.	**Aconite 30c.** One dose and repeat as necessary.
Anxiety; sweating. 'Running to the toilet'. Hurried in everything.	**Argentum Nitricum 30c.** One dose and repeat as necessary.
Anxious, restless; fastidious. Fear of death. Worse at 2 a.m.	**Arsenicum Album 30c.** One dose and repeat as necessary.
Anxiety; weakness of muscles. Trembling; 'butterflies in tummy'.	**Gelsemium 30c.** One dose and repeat as necessary.

COMING UP TO CONFINEMENT – last days

To reduce bruising of the tissues, and to curtail bleeding.	**Arnica 6c** or **30c.** At onset of labour pains and three times a day during and after confinement for 3–5 days.
To allay the pain and discomfort of colicky contractions of the womb.	**Caulophyllum 6c.** One dose, at intervals of one to two hours, for 2–4 doses.
To reduce the pain of 'cuts' and the injury to nerve endings.	**Hypericum 6c.** At onset of labour pains and three times a day during and after confinement for 1–2 days.

Take the Arnica and Hypericum together, as it may not be possible to remember to take them separately.

AFTER THE CONFINEMENT

Shock; excitement; fear; sleeplessness. Unable to pass urine.	**Aconite 30c.** One dose as soon as possible and repeat thirty minutes later if necessary.
Sore, bruised; bed feels hard; aches all over. Very tired.	**Arnica 6c** or **30c.** One dose as soon as possible after the birth, and three times a day for 3–5 days.
Slow labour with much stretching. Overstretched bladder. Unable to pass urine.	**Causticum 6c.** One dose and repeat thirty minutes later if necessary.
'Cuts' (episiotomy)	**Hypericum 6c.** One dose, three to four times a day, for 2–3 days.
After catheterisation, overstretching.	**Staphysagria 6c.** One dose, three times a day, for 2–3 days.

External Treatment

In order to bathe the line of stitches after being cut (episiotomy), or torn: make up a fresh solution of **Calendula** or **Hypercal** 5ml (20 drops) to 200ml (half a pint) of previously boiled and cooled water.

Breastfeeding Problems

TOO LITTLE MILK

Loss of milk. Breasts decrease in size. Thirsty and depressed.

Lac Defloratum 6c. One dose, 2–3 times a day, and reduce with improvement.

Milk scanty. Nursing painful, radiating to chest and neck. Mother tearful and moping. Feels worse with a hot, stuffy room. Wants fresh air.

Pulsatilla 6c. One dose, 2–3 times a day, and reduce with improvement.

TOO MUCH MILK

Free flow of milk. Breasts swollen and inflamed, and very tender; red, hot and hard. Mother flushed and hot. Skin hot and dry.

Belladonna 6c. One dose every 2–4 hours until settled.

Free flow of watery milk. Baby refuses and cries. Breasts swollen. Patient chilly and anxious; perspires on head and face.

Calcarea Carbonica 6c. One dose, three times a day, for 3–5 days and reduce.

Free flow of milk. Breasts hard and lumpy. Nipples very sore. Nursing very painful – pain radiates all over body.

Phytolacca 6c. One dose, 2–3 times a day, reducing with improvement.

SORE NIPPLES

Nipples very inflamed and tender; too painful to nurse. Mother very irritable and intolerant of the pain. Worse at night and with heat.

Chamomilla 6c. One dose every 30 minutes to 1 hour. Reduce with improvement

Nipples cracked, very sensitive; splinter-like pains.

Nitric Acid 6c. One dose every 30 minutes to 1 hour. Reduce with improvement.

Generally very chilly – especially hands and feet. Nipples very sore, ulcerating easily. May be indrawn.

Silica 6c or **30c.** One dose every 2–4 hours. Reduce with improvement.

Painful flow of milk, impossible to start nursing. Emotional upsets; broody and moody. Resentful, ill-tempered and oversensitive.

Staphysagria 6c or **30c.** One dose every 2–4 hours. Reduce with improvement.

External Treatment – apply **Hypercal** cream to nipples between feeds.

INFLAMMATION OF BREASTS (MASTITIS)

This is a common problem during breastfeeding. It starts as a general flu-like feeling, with a fever and aches and pains throughout the body. At this stage the breasts may not be particularly painful, but if inspected, one may detect a reddened area on one of the breasts with underlying tenderness. Homoeopathic remedies used at this stage are extremely efficacious and often eliminate the need for antibiotics. However, if the reddened area increases, together with pain and fever, the doctor must be consulted the same day.

- It is important to *continue* to breastfeed during the episode of mastitis, in order to empty the breast. The milk will not be harmful to the baby.
- Homoeopathic medicine are absolutely safe during breastfeeding.

Throbbing or hot stinging pain. Breasts feel heavy and hard; streaks radiate from nipple. Worse with touch, jarring and lying down. Better semi-erect. Swelling – early abscess formation. May be a fever.

Belladonna 6c or **30c.** One dose every 2 hours. Reduce with improvement.

Milk fever and breast abscesses. Breasts hot, painful and hard. Small knotty lumps – very sore. Tearing pains with movement. Worse for warmth, motion and touch. Better for pressure and lying on painful side.

Bryonia 6c or **30c.** One dose every 2 hours. Reduce with improvement.

Breasts hard, painful and blue coloured. Abscess formation. Cracks and smaller ulcers around nipples. When nursing, pain goes from nipple all over body.

Phytolacca 6c or **30c.** One dose every 2 hours. Reduce with improvement.

Menopause ('Change of Life')

The menopause occurs when the periods cease, but the problems associated with it all too frequently develop before this time and can extend beyond it.

These problems arise because of hormone imbalance. The symptoms vary greatly in their complexity and severity, as does the length of time needed by the body to create a new balance.

However, in the background of a woman's life at this time there may be emotional conflicts which arise for entirely different reasons. There may, for example, be marital disharmony, or children may be leaving the family home. Aged parents may also be causing emotional and physical stress.

It is clear that the difficulties a woman may experience at this time of her life are likely to be the complex interworking of many factors from several sources. It is unlikely that simply giving hormone replacement therapy will be enough. By the same token, it is not enough to treat the emotional problems alone. Homoeopathic remedies are especially valuable in these circumstances in that they act upon the physical and mental aspects of the individual patient.

When a woman becomes aware that she has started the change of life, it is essential that she has the benefit of a cervical smear test, internal examination, breast examination and so on, even if she has no symptoms that worry her.

If the medical investigations are all clear, but the remedies below have not been helpful, you should read the other sections in this part of the book to form an extended and more accurate picture. However, if none of the remedies indicated provide relief it may be the result of homoeopathic over-simplication. In these circumstances my advice is to consult an experienced homoeopath for a full evaluation.

HOT FLUSHES

Hot flushes of the head and face: redness and congestion; sudden start and finish; profuse sweating of face.	**Belladonna 6c.** One dose at fifteen minute intervals for 3–4 doses.
Hot flushes of the head and face: as above *and* rapid palpitations of the heart.	**Glonoinum 6c.** One dose at fifteen minute intervals for 3–4 doses.
Red-faced, irritable, angry, talkative, jealous, suspicious. Worse – morning and after sleep, from heat and alcohol, from tight clothes. Better – in cool air.	**Lachesis 30c***
Gentle and weepy, changeable moods, needs sympathy and reassurance. Worse – heat and humidity; tight clothes. Better – gentle exercise and fresh air.	**Pulsatilla 30c***
Sallow-faced, irritable, weepy, angry, depressed; loss of sexual urge; low, dragging backache. Worse – evening, extreme cold or humidity. Better – for fresh air, sleep, vigorous exercise or dancing.	**Sepia 30c***

*Three possible dosage schemes for Lachesis, Sepia and Pulsatilla:

- One dose morning, evening and the following morning, starting on day twelve of the menstrual cycle.
- One dose morning and evening for one or two days a week.
- One dose when needed.

See overleaf for other problems associated with the menopause.

OTHER PROBLEMS ASSOCIATED WITH THE MENOPAUSE

There are other problems which can occur during the change of life. Some of these are not just menopausal and are dealt with elsewhere in this book. Some of the more particularly menopausal problems may not be 'important' from the medical point of view. However, they do make day-to-day life unpleasant and can add up to a situation affecting the woman's family and friends.

Simple measures may do away with much of the chronic low grade 'illness' of this age group. Homoeopathic remedies can be used to eliminate or reduce the need for hormones, tranquillisers, antidepressants and sleeping pills.

Fatigue, exhaustion. Aching muscles, backache. Tired, aching legs. Bruising and discolouration. Small 'burst veins'.	**Arnica 6c**
Arthritic pains in small joints, especially fingers. Nervous tension and anxiety, emotional instability.	**Caulophyllum 6c**
Timid, sad, indecisive, emotional and weepy with music, not interested in sex.	**Graphites 30c**
Varicose veins. Swollen, tender veins. Aching and stiffness.	**Hamamelis 6c**
Nervous and depressed. Frequent sighing, exaggerated responses, contrary emotions. Areas of numbness. Lump in the throat.	**Ignatia 30c**

Dosage: One dose 2–3 times each day, reducing the frequency with improvement.

CHILDREN'S PROBLEMS

Homoeopathy is particularly helpful for the problems of children, in part because they are not generally troubled by the after-effects of repeated illnesses, or previous medical treatment, or by the build-up of chemicals from modern diets.

Remember that children fluctuate alarmingly in their symptoms in a few hours ('Up one minute and down the next'), so do not panic.

Check the circumstances and the symptoms against those given in the following pages, and find the most appropriate remedy. Then give it to the child as suggested.

But remember too that babies can become more seriously unwell at a quicker rate than older children and adults. For example, a baby with diarrhoea can dehydrate rapidly in hot weather, as can a young child with an acute tonsillitis who refuses to drink because of the pain.

Homoeopathic remedies may be given to a baby as a powder. If no powders are available, the remedy in pill or tablet form may be crushed between two clean, dry teaspoons. The powder is then placed in the mouth of the baby, or dissolved in a tablespoonful of water: feed one teaspoonful per dose.

This method can be used if several doses of a remedy need to be given through the day and night.

If you have any doubts about any situation, it is essential that you consult your own doctor immediately.

The Newborn Baby

AFTER DELIVERY

Most babies are delivered quite normally without any undue problems, but occasionally the mother's labour is either prolonged or very rapid. For some reason, forceps may have to be used. In all these circumstances the baby's head will have had 'a rough passage', and homoeopathic remedies will help the bruising which may have resulted.

Particularly after a prolonged labour or a forceps delivery, or for bruising and swelling.	**Arnica 6c** or **30c** **Calendula 6c**

Dosage: Take these two remedies together, one dose of each three times a day for 3 days.

SOFT TISSUE SWELLING OF THE SCALP

Soft tissue swelling of the baby's scalp (caput) is normal and usually disappears in two or three days. If it persists after using Arnica and Calendula, use the other remedies, and consult your own doctor.

Soft tissue swelling of the baby's scalp which persists for more than 2–3 days.	**Calcarea Carbonica 6c.** One dose morning and evening for 3 days, *or* **Silica 6c.** One dose morning and evening for 3 days.

HERNIA

A hernia is a swelling of the local area of the wall of the tummy, frequently around the naval. Hernias protrude when the baby cries but usually they are not as serious as they look, and most disappear of their own accord.

Most hernias disappear in a few weeks. Leave them, or try:	**Nux Vomica 6c.** One dose twice a week for 1 month.

JAUNDICE

This yellow colouration occurs in most, if not all, newborn white babies, and is quite natural. It usually becomes apparent on the second or third day after delivery and fades away two or three days after. **If the yellow discolouration deepens or continues, consult your doctor.**

A mild yellowing of the skin for 2–3 days in a white baby is normal.	**China 6c.** One dose morning and evening for 4–5 days.

SWOLLEN BREASTS

Do nothing. This is very common, and they will go down in a few days. **Do not squeeze.**

If anyone has squeezed the swollen breast.	**Arnica 6c** or **30c.** Two doses a day for 2–3 days.

CONJUNCTIVITIS ('STICKY EYES')

Babies born in hospital commonly have eyes which discharge yellow pus. The cause is contamination by germs which are increasingly resistant to antibiotics. It is important to clean the eyes of the baby two or three times a day as follows:

Using a small swab of sterile cotton wool, which has been moistened with cooled, boiled water, apply gentle pressure to the inner corner of the eye and gently sweep outwards. Discard the swab and repeat the action. If necessary, use the same procedure with the other eye, using new swabs.

Yellow or white discharge. Pinkness of the whites of the eyes. *Use this first.*	**Argentum Nitricum 6c.** One dose every four hours for 2–3 days.
Profuse discharge of bland white or yellow pus.	**Pulsatilla 6c.** One dose every four hours for 3–4 days.
Later, 'stickiness' of the lids, especially in the morning.	**Calcarea Carbonica 6c.** One dose three times a day for 3–4 days.

If there is no improvement after three days, **seek medical advice**.

The Baby

FEEDING PROBLEMS

Breastfeeding is almost always best; there can be very few situations when this is not so.

The mother's milk provides the factors which defend the baby against infections before it has any immunity of its own. At the same time, the mother's milk provides the baby with the food which nature intended it to have.

There seems to be little doubt that, however carefully cows' milk is treated to make it as near as possible to maternal milk, the proteins within it remain foreign material. This may result in babies developing eczema and asthma, especially in families which have a history of allergies in general.

Milk Intolerance

This may be due to poor feeding techniques, but it may also be genuine intolerance. In this case seek advice, but do not go from one brand of powdered milk to the other needlessly.

Wind and Colic

Colic can occur without wind, and a rumbling, windy tummy need not give rise to colic. Colic is a pain tending to come and go. The baby may twist about and draw its legs up at the height of the pain.

The problem is very common, but if it continues for two or three hours, or if the baby is obviously distressed, call your doctor. A rare condition occurs when the baby suffers increasingly frequent and severe attacks of colic. It draws up its legs and cries with the pain and then falls asleep, pale and shocked-looking. The baby may then pass a loose motion with some bright red blood ('redcurrant jelly stool'). **It is vital to call the doctor immediately or else to take the baby to hospital immediately.**

FEEDING PROBLEMS

Milk Intolerance

Great anguish; vomits everything; falls asleep after vomiting. Violent straining and thin, green, undigested stool.	**Aethusa 6c.** Three doses a day until improvement.
Chilly, fat baby with a large head. Sweats about the head; is pale and flabby; teething delayed. Chalky stools.	**Calcarea Carbonica 6c.** Three doses a day until improvement.
Rejects milk, which causes diarrhoea. Swollen abdomen with loud rumbling of painful wind.	**Natrum Carbonicum 6c.** Three doses a day until improvement.

Wind and Colic

Tummy blown up. Wind passed in small quantities with no relief, improved by warmth. Not much better when picked up. Irritable and obviously in pain.	**Chamomilla 6c.** One dose every half hour for up to 3 doses. Repeat when necessary.
Writhing and twisting. Cannot keep still; better passing wind; may be caused by anger.	**Colocynthis 6c.** One dose every half hour for up to 3 doses. Repeat when necessary.
Chilly, irritable, angry. Overfeeding.	**Nux Vomica 6c.** One dose every half hour for up to 3 doses. Repeat when necessary.
'Three month colic'. Whining and windy, vomiting, perhaps rejecting the milk. Pitiful crying, stops on being picked up.	**Pulsatilla 6c.** One dose every half hour for up to 3 doses. Repeat when necessary.

If the condition recurs, or at any time the symptoms are severe and no relief is obtained by homoeopathic remedies, consult your doctor.

DIARRHOEA

This may be the result of bowel infection or intolerance to a particular food, if it occurs acutely. If there are recurrences, it may be due to alterations in feeding such as weaning. Teething or infections of the throat, nose or chest can also give rise to diarrhoea.

If there is an infection of any of these areas, turn to the appropriate page in the children's section and treat the condition. It is only then that the diarrhoea is likely to subside.

Remember that a baby may lose body fluids rapidly ('dehydration') and become seriously ill. This will be worse if the baby has a high temperature, is vomiting or not taking liquids or milk, or if the weather is hot. Do not hesitate to call your own doctor or take the baby to hospital if improvement does not begin in under a day.

DIARRHOEA ALTERNATING WITH CONSTIPATION

This is only likely to occur over a period of several days or even weeks, so that there is no urgency. However, attention must be paid to the general health and to the diet and liquid intake, and you should seek the advice of your doctor or the health visitor. In addition, a homoeopath may well decide to treat the baby constitutionally.

DIARRHOEA

Pallor with white upper lip. Facial anxiety and pain. Vomiting after milk. Motion undigested, thin and green. Drowsy – not restless.	**Aethusa 6c.** One dose every 2–4 hours. Stop with improvement.
Stools painless, very smelly and watery. Vomiting and diarrhoea together. Rapid dehydration possible. Very restless. Very thirsty.	**Arsenicum Album 6c.** One dose every 2–4 hours. Stop with improvement.
Fretful baby, crying and only ceasing when held close. Legs drawn up. Slimy, watery green stool which smells like rotten eggs. Anus red and raw. Yellow stool turns green on exposure to air.	**Chamomilla 6c.** One dose every 2–4 hours. Stop with improvement.
Jets of yellow, watery motion brought on by feeding.	**Croton Tiglium 6c.** One dose every 2–4 hours. Stop with improvement.
Pale face, crying. Vomiting. Clean mouth and tongue. Stools putrid-smelling.	**Ipecacuanha 6c.** One dose every 2–4 hours. Stop with improvement.
Chilly, shivering baby. Stools copious, sour-smelling. Colicky pains and wind. Great straining with stool. May have profuse salivation and mouth ulcers.	**Mercurius Solubilis 6c.** One dose every 2–4 hours. Stop with improvement.

DIARRHOEA ALTERNATING WITH CONSTIPATION

Frequently happens in warm weather.	**Bryonia 6c.** One dose three times a day for 3–5 days.
Perhaps with undigested food particles. Can occur in cold weather and is better in warmth.	**Nux Vomica 6c.** One dose three times a day for 3–5 days.

NAPPY RASH

This is a common skin condition, usually caused by germs in the nappy and on the skin in the nappy area. These germs break down the urine to form ammonia, which is the actual chemical cause of the rash. Detergents which are not rinsed out of nappies are also another cause.

Prevention really consists of thoroughly washing nappies and rinsing several times, with the last rinsing water containing a mild antiseptic which is dried into the nappy. An alternative practice is to use a disposable nappy.

Do *not* keep a wet or dirty nappy on the baby.

Treatment of the rash consists of allowing fresh air to get to the skin as much as conditions allow, giving the skin a chance to dry. Use bland creams or ointments before putting on the nappy. The traditional 'Zinc and Castor Oil' is generally most acceptable, but there may be individual preferences.

TEETHING

There are twenty milk teeth (baby teeth), and the first to appear at about six to ten months are the lower incisors. The last to appear are the second molars, from twenty to thirty months. A few children are born with teeth, while others do not produce the first teeth until after the first birthday. There is a very wide variation in normal children.

Most babies suffer discomfort or actual pain when teething, and produce large quantities of saliva. Gnawing and chewing on rusks or teething rings seems to give comfort. Redness around the mouth and chin will be helped by applying **Calendula** cream or ointment.

The remedies on the opposite page will help to ease the pain and general malaise. For pain with inflammation see page 157.

Other conditions such as ear infections, colds and chesty coughs occur coincidentally and are not caused by the teething. However, some babies do seem to become 'chesty' with each erupting tooth. Check the remedies for 'Cough' (pages 87 and 126–7), and 'Colds and Influenza' (pages 84–5, 120–3 and 158–9).

NAPPY RASH

Chilly baby, fat and flabby. Better when warm. Sweating head at night.	**Calcarea Carbonica 6c.** One dose three times a day. Stop with improvement.
Hot baby; red skin worse in the heat. Worse for bathing; better in the fresh air.	**Sulphur 6c.** One dose every day. Stop with improvement.

TEETHING

Chilly, fat and flabby. Sweating head at night. Especially useful when dentition is delayed.	**Calcarea Carbonica 6c.** One dose three times a day. Stop with improvement.
Chilly, but thinner and wiry.	**Calcarea Phosphorica 6c.** One dose three times a day. Stop with improvement.
Very painful. Intense irritability. Can't be settled down. Angry, and helped by carrying. Diarrhoea – green, offensive smell. Often has one red and one pale cheek.	**Chamomilla 6c.** One dose three times a day. Stop with improvement.

THE CRYING BABY

The first thing to do is to check what is wrong or, indeed, if anything is wrong at all:

- Is there a fever?
- Does the baby look ill?
- Does the nappy need changing?
- Has the baby passed a motion? Is it loose and offensive?
- Does the baby need feeding?

See other pages in this section for conditions such as teething, colic, diarrhoea, etc.

CONVULSIONS (FITS)

The baby usually has an infection with a high temperature which affects the working of the brain. The fit normally shows itself as a twitching of the face, arms and legs and occasionally the whole body. The breath is held and the skin becomes deep red and then a blotchy purple. After a few seconds the twitching stops, the breathing restarts and the baby becomes pink again.

All of this is alarming to the parents, but usually fits look worse than they are.

The first steps are:

1) Remain calm.
2) Unclothe the baby.
3) Cool it down by bathing it in tepid water.
4) At the same time give the remedy indicated.

If the baby does not settle down or if further fits occur, **call the doctor now**. If the condition settles, consult the doctor at the first suitable time.

THE CRYING BABY

Whining and rejecting. Doesn't want to be picked up. Worse for touching.	**Antimonium Crudum 6c.** One dose and repeat if necessary at fifteen minute intervals for up to 4 doses.
Angry, excitable, irritable, lashes out. Inconsolable. Wants to be carried about constantly. Cries when put down.	**Chamomilla 6c.** One dose and repeat if necessary at fifteen minute intervals for up to 4 doses.
Angry, oversensitive. Chilly; better for warmth.	**Nux Vomica 6c.** One dose and repeat if necessary at fifteen minute intervals for up to 4 doses.
Whimpering, 'whingeing', stops when cuddled. Wants affection.	**Pulsatilla 6c.** One dose and repeat if necessary at fifteen minute intervals for up to 4 doses.

CONVULSIONS (FITS)

Hot, red with fever. Dilated pupils.	**Belladonna 6c.** One dose and repeat in fifteen minutes if necessary. Continue every two to three hours for 1–2 days, to treat the underlying infection.
Teething. Extremely agitated; violently restless.	**Chamomilla 6c.** One dose and repeat in fifteen minutes if necessary.
After fright.	**Ignatia 6c.** One dose and repeat in fifteen minutes if necessary.
Anger and irritation.	**Nux Vomica 6c.** One dose and repeat in fifteen minutes if necessary.

Toddlers and School Children

ADENOIDS – LARGE

(Nasal voice, mouth breathing, snoring, dull hearing or intermittent deafness.)

This condition frequently occurs with a cold, and sometimes with acute tonsillitis. Usually when the immediate illness subsides, so do the adenoids; but not always. In this case a long-term problem arises.

Remember that it may be necessary for the child's wellbeing to use antibiotics in certain circumstances, and their use should not be spurned out of hand. However, repeated doses of antibiotics are not helpful. Antihistamines and drying agents also give rise to many problems. They may help in the short term, but if used at all should only be used very sparingly.

While it is true that this situation settles down by about the age of 10 or 11 years, an awful lot of trouble can arise before then. The general poor health and unhappiness and the loss of school time worries parents.

The use of homoeopathic remedies in the sudden, acute stages can be very helpful.

Another way of using remedies is to 'build up the resistance' of the child. This is probably best done after thoughtful enquiry into the family background by a homoeopath.

ADENOIDS – LARGE

Constant mouth breathing. Tonsils and neck glands enlarged. Poorly developing child both mentally and physically.	**Baryta Carbonica 6c.** One dose twice a day for 10–14 days.
Green-yellow catarrh. Mouth breathing. Squelching in the ears with dull hearing. Whining and wants to be cuddled. Can be better in fresh air.	**Pulsatilla 6c.** One dose twice a day for 10–14 days.
Snuffling, snoring. Glands in throat and neck swollen. Swallowing difficult. Feels the cold, catches cold easily.	**Silica 6c.** One dose twice a day for 10–14 days.

All these short courses of treatment may have to be repeated if the symptoms return.

ASTHMA IN CHILDREN

A child with a history of asthma may well have episodes of tightness of the chest and wheezy breathlessness, but sometimes only a tight repetitive cough which escapes notice and diagnosis. It can be brought on by colds and chest infections, inhaling cold air, exercise, and by contact with allergens such as cat fur, dog hair, horse hair, feathers and house dust.

If a cause such as an allergy can be established, preventative measures can be used:

- Avoid contact with the particular cause, and . . .
- Use a homoeopathic remedy made from the particular allergen.

The first signs of asthma in children can be:

- Chest infections following frequent colds and upper respiratory infections.
- A repetitive cough instead of wheezing, especially in very young children.
- Breathlessness in cold weather when not exercising.

If you are suddenly faced with a child with breathing problems, either call your doctor or take the child to the nearest hospital with an Accident & Emergency Department. (But check where this is first – not all hospitals have one. You will find the numbers in the phone book under 'Hospitals'.) Whilst waiting for medical help the remedies on the opposite page can be tried.

Asthma in childhood can be treated effectively by homoeopathy, but this should be done under the care of a qualified practitioner. It is important that the child continues with the conventional medication prescribed by the doctor. Homoeopathy is used here in a complementary way.

ASTHMA IN CHILDREN

Asthma after fit of anger. Irritable hard, dry cough. Better from bending head backwards; cold, fresh air and drinking cold water; and being carried about. Impatient, irritable and whining; spiteful.	**Chamomilla 30c.** One dose every 15–30 minutes. Reduce with improvement.
Asthmatic bronchitis – rattling and bubbling. Chest full of mucus – but not easily coughed up. Better sitting up to breathe; better in open air or by open windows. Spasmodic coughing violently with each breath till blue in the face. Nausea and gagging and much saliva. Hoarseness at end of episode. Returns periodically each year.	**Ipecacuanha 6c** or **30c.** One dose every 15–30 minutes. Reduce with improvement.
Worse 4 to 5 a.m. and in cold, wet weather and cold, damp places. Very breathless, with much rattling of mucus in chest. Mucus thick and greenish. Pain in lower chest. Every cold results in asthma.	**Natrum Sulphuricum 6c** or **30c.** One dose every 15–30 minutes. Reduce with improvement.
Great difficulty breathing or lying down. Variable hoarseness. Dry cough early night, loose cough in the morning – yellow green sticky mucus. Better open air and gentle motion, sympathy and consolation. Worse for heat of a warm room.	**Pulsatilla 6c** or **30c.** One dose every 15–30 minutes. Reduce with improvement.
Attacks of asthma about 3 a.m. – suddenly. Gasping for breath; turns blue. Better sitting up – improves and falls asleep. Cycle then repeated. Noise. Blocked nose. Can breathe in but not out. (See section on 'Croup', pages 88–9).	**Sambucus 6c** or **30c.** One dose every 15–30 minutes. Reduce with improvement.

Refer also to the sections on: 'Coughs and Colds', pages 87 and 126–7; and 'Influenza', pages 158–9.

BEDWETTING

Bedwetting occurs when the control of the bladder is lost during sleep and urine is passed unconsciously. Some children may never have developed bladder control at night.

Other children may be incontinent during the day also. This may be due to 'being lazy' – they may be far more interested in what they are doing, and rush to the toilet too late. Usually it is best to train the child to use the toilet at fairly regular intervals.

A far smaller group of children may leak fairly constantly all day and all night. These children need to be taken to the family doctor for possible investigation into the anatomy and nervous control of the bladder.

By far the largest group of children simply 'wet the bed'. If the child is sensitive and anxious, the cause may be obvious and the treatment is to support and to encourage the sufferer. This will reduce the bedwetting and the source of anxiety.

If the problem persists in any of these forms, ask the family doctor if the child might be referred to the Continence Adviser.

General Management

- Sympathy and encouragement, and a praise instead of blame approach is best. Ignore wet nights but give 'stars' for the dry nights.
- The incontinence pad with an alarm bell may help the deep sleepers, and can be arranged by your own doctor and health visitor.
- Avoid giving the child large drinks in the late evening and before going to bed.
- Arrange for the child to use the toilet three times before bedtime, say half an hour, a quarter of an hour and immediately before getting into bed.
- Arrange for either parent to 'lift' the drowsy or sleeping child to the toilet when they go to bed themselves.

Whilst doing all or any of these things, use homoeopathic remedies as an aid. However, for many of these children bedwetting may be a problem of long duration. If these remedies are not helpful, seek the advice of an experienced homoeopath.

BEDWETTING

May be wet during the day also. Leaks with coughing. Wet early in sleep; not aware of passing urine. Irritable and very sensitive to cold.

Causticum 6c. One dose 6 times a day for 5–10 days. With improvement, reduce to one dose before bedtime.

Frequency during the day. 'Soaks the bed'. Dream and nightmares. Dull discomfort and tenderness in the bladder. (Consult the doctor about possible bladder infection.)

Equisetum 6c. One dose 4–6 times a day for 5–10 days. With improvement, reduce to one dose before bedtime.

'Soaks the bed' later in sleep. Irritable, peevish and fretful. Worse on waking. Hates contradiction. Likes fresh air.

Lycopodium 30c. One dose before bedtime for 5–10 days.

Debility after recent illness or recent growth spurt or overtaxed at school. Listless and apathetic. Profuse milky urine. Anxiety first, burning after.

Phosphoric Acid 6c or **30c.** One dose before bedtime for 5–10 days.

Large quantities of urine. 'Soaks the bed' early in sleep.

Plantago 6c or **30c.** One dose before bedtime for 5–10 days.

Increased need to pass urine. Worse lying down and coughing. Very changeable; timid and likes sympathy and cuddles.

Pulsatilla 6c or **30c.** One dose before bedtime for 5–10 days.

Urgency – can't wait – doesn't wake up in time. Untidy warm-blooded children. Thirsty and craves sweets.

Sulphur 6c or **30c.** One dose before bedtime for 5–10 days.

COLDS AND INFLUENZA IN CHILDREN

Not much can be done to prevent children from being exposed to viral infections at school. Indeed, their first years at school are frequently a long succession of infections.

If the child is basically healthy there is little to worry about, since children benefit from developing immunity to all the germs they encounter. Each illness can be satisfactorily dealt with using homoeopathic remedies, as indicated by the patient's symptoms, and each illness can be regarded as a necessary stepping stone to maturity.

The problem arises when the child goes from one illness to the next without ever recovering properly. They can be made to feel even worse by the prescription of antibiotics. In this situation the use of 'Cold and Flu tablets' (made up by the major homoeopathic manufacturers), taken at monthly intervals around the year, can be very effective in reversing the trend.

Prevention

A good diet is essential, with a plentiful supply of fresh fruit and vegetables.

Additional vitamins, especially vitamin C during and after illness, should be taken in the quantities recommended by the particular manufacturer. Many people believe that extra vitamin C prevents infections. It may do so, and the fact that scientists have not proved the matter one way or the other need not prevent you from playing safe.

Children need plenty of exercise, and should take enough to become healthily tired. They should be in the open air as much as possible, exposed to sunshine, care being taken to avoid overexposure and sunburn.

Treatment

- Use the homoeopathic remedies as indicated by the main symptoms of the patient, changing them as the picture changes, if necessary.
- Rest the child, preferably in bed, but downstairs if it will not settle easily. The room should be light and airy; the patient should not be overclothed and allowed to become too hot.
- The child should be encouraged to drink as much as possible.
- Remember that as the child recovers, it will need toys and games and puzzles to occupy its mind. Try to avoid the hypnotic effect of too much television.

COLDS AND INFLUENZA IN CHILDREN

Refer to the following sections for advice on particular remedies: 'Colds', pages 120–3; 'Fevers', pages 96–103; 'Influenza', pages 158–9; and 'Sore Throat', pages 196–7.

Prevention

'Cold and Flu tablets'. One dose morning and evening on the first day of each month through the year, and perhaps every two weeks during the winter.

This method of prevention should be continued only until the child has obviously improved in general health, and has not had bad colds, sore throats, catarrh and ear problems during the previous winter. If they have been successfully treated, a cold will have been short-lived and recovery complete.

Chesty Cold

In some children a cold always 'goes on to the chest'. There is often a family tendency to respond in this way. In this case, constitutional treatment by an experienced homoeopath is likely to eradicate the tendency.

CONSTIPATION IN CHILDREN

General Management

- Encourage the child to use the toilet at regular times, but do not cause resentment or anxiety in the process.
- Train the child to go to the toilet as soon as the urge to empty the bowels occurs. This is easier said than done, especially when the child is reading, playing or watching TV.
- Drinking adequate quantities of water will help to prevent the motions from becoming hard. Remember that the child will require more drinks in very hot weather, or if it is unwell with a high temperature.
- Increase the amount of fibre in the diet. This is best done by giving wholemeal bread and cereals, and by increasing the quantity of fruit and vegetables eaten daily. At the same time eliminate the highly refined and manufactured foods. In short – cut out 'junk food' and provide a wholefood diet.

Straining for a soft sticky stool. Unable to pass stool until a large accumulation. Older children who eat indigestible things.	**Alumina 6c.** One dose two to three times a day. Stop with improvement.
In chilly, sedentary children with sluggish bowel action. Feels better when constipated.	**Calçarea Carbonica 6c.** One dose morning and evening. Stop with improvement.
Frequent and ineffectual desire. Small quantities at each attempt. Alternating with diarrhoea. Impatient and oversensitive.	**Nux Vomica 6c.** One dose morning and evening. Stop with improvement.
No desire for stool. No complaints. Bowels seem closed.	**Opium 6c.** One dose morning and evening. Stop with improvement.

COUGH IN CHILDREN

Refer also to the following sections: 'Cough' (in adults), pages 126–7 and 'Croup' (overleaf).

General Measures

It is usually wise to keep the patient indoors in a warm, airy room if the weather is bad, and to avoid changes in temperature or places where the cough is worsened, in order to prevent fresh outbursts of coughing.

Check the symptoms of the patient and choose the most suitable remedy in the sections mentioned above.

Call the doctor if:

- The overall condition worsens.
- The child has other medical problems.
- Progress is not being made in a reasonable time – say three or four days.

Sometimes coughs can drag on for weeks. In other cases, the child may have repeated infections over a period of years. In both these situations the child can be said to have a basic weakness, and this can only be treated on constitutional grounds. Such treatment is beyond the scope of this book and you should consult an experienced homoeopath.

CROUP

This is a spasm of the vocal cords which makes *breathing in* difficult, giving a sensation of suffocation. It usually occurs at night. The child may already have a cough or a cold, but it can come 'out of the blue'. It causes a crowing or croaking noise, frequently with a barking or metallic cough.

All this makes the child and the parents frightened, which again aggravates the problem, creating a vicious circle of spasm, breathing difficulty, and fear.

The attack may last from one to three hours and then rapidly ease off, but it can recur for two or three nights.

Croup can be dangerous and should not be ignored.

Treatment – General Measures

- Be **calm** and **soothing** and **reassuring**.
- Handle the child gently. Sitting up is usually the best position but cuddle the child in its favourite position.
- Use the homoeopathic remedies listed on the opposite page.
- Create a warm, moist atmosphere in the room, using a steadily steaming kettle to help with this.

Note the condition of the child. **Call your doctor** if there are no obvious signs of improvement in 30–60 minutes, or if at any time the spasm worsens or the breathing becomes difficult, or if the colour of the lips and fingernails of the child turns blue.

CROUP

Take in order:

Use at the early stage of any fever but especially to allay fear. Use first in croup.	**Aconite 30c**
Can also be helpful in suffocating coughing spells. Worse in cold atmosphere. Worse with cold draughts.	**Hepar Sulphuris 30c** or **6c**
Can also be helpful for the child who wakes from sleep, choking with a violent cough.	**Spongia 30c** or **6c**

Dosage: The recognised treatment for croup is first to give a dose of Aconite 30c, followed in ten to fifteen minutes by Hepar Sulphuris 30c and by Spongia 30c ten to fifteen minutes after that. Then return to the Hepar Sulphuris, continuing the treatment as required by alternating Hepar Sulphuris with Spongia at ten to fifteen minute intervals. Use whatever potency is available, but the 30c is likely to be more powerful.

EARACHE

This is usually caused by infection behind the eardrum, having developed from infection of the throat and nasal passages. The eardrum becomes inflamed and painful. Pus may form behind the eardrum, increasing the pressure and forcing the drum to bulge outwards. This increases the pain. At the same time the child becomes very unwell and 'toxic' with a fever.

If homoeopathic remedies appropriate to the particular child are used quickly, the whole sequence may be stopped, and the child will recover quickly.

Most ear infections are due to viruses and usually clear within 48 hours. If not, then consult your doctor.

If the above situation is a one-off event and the treatment suggested is successful, then that is the end of the matter. But if the earache is repeated several times each winter, or forms part of a picture of frequent colds and chest infections, there is an underlying constitutional weakness which can only be helped by 'constitutional' treatment. You must consult an experienced homoeopath for this.

EARACHE

Abrupt onset of pain in ear, especially after a chill in cold, dry weather. Unbearable and usually worse at night, some improvement by local heat; skin burning and dry; fever with shivering. Anxious and restless, fearful.

Aconite 30c. One dose at intervals of thirty minutes for 3–4 doses. If no improvement, move on to one of the other remedies.

Pain, stinging, burning, pricking. External ear may be red and tender. Eased by cold compresses; made worse by heat. Hot dry skin alternating with perspiration.

Apis 6c. One dose at intervals of thirty minutes and reduce with improvement.

Throbbing pain, not so rapid onset. Very hot dry skin, red face and dilated pupils. Not restless or fearful.

Belladonna 6c. One dose at intervals of thirty minutes and reduce with improvement.

Stabbing pain, intolerable. Cross, irritable; doesn't know where to put himself.

Chamomilla 6c. One dose at intervals of thirty minutes and reduce with improvement.

Jerking, tearing pain, ears hot. Pain is made worse by heat. Miserable and whining; responds to cuddling and affection.

Pulsatilla 6c. One dose at intervals of thirty minutes and reduce with improvement.

EARS – DISCHARGING

Discharge may arise from the walls of the canal leading down from the outer ear to the eardrum. But it is safer to remember that it can arise from the bursting of the eardrum by the pressure of pus behind it.

Earache which ceases suddenly followed by the appearance of pus discharging from the ear canal probably means that the eardrum has burst. This is not an emergency because the pressure in the ear has been relieved – when the infection has subsided with treatment the eardrum will heal. The perforation will close and hearing will return to normal.

Use homoeopathic remedies which may already be helping, or change to a remedy which is indicated by the type of pus being discharged.

For ears which have discharged many times – chronic ears – it would be better to consult an experienced homoeopath.

It may be necessary to use antibiotics. If this course is decided upon, it will be helpful to use homoeopathic remedies at the same time.

FLUID IN THE EARS ('GLUE EAR')

This usually occurs after ear infections following a cold. It may only last a few days, but it may take many weeks to clear. Your doctor should be consulted if deafness or poor hearing persists, in order that the level of hearing can be monitored.

EARS – DISCHARGING

Yellow pus – flows easily. Very sensitive to draughts.	**Hepar Sulphuris 6c.** One dose three times a day until improvement.
Thick, white, stringy pus; very sticky and difficult to clean.	**Kali Muriaticum 6c.** One dose three times a day until improvement.
Yellow-green pus; thicker, sticky.	**Pulsatilla 6c.** One dose three times a day until improvement.
Foul-smelling pus.	**Pyrogen 6c.** One dose three times a day until improvement.

When the discharge stops, continue the original treatment for two further days, and then give **Sulphur 6c** morning and evening for two days more.

If ear, nose and throat infections are promptly and correctly treated, 'glue ear' is not likely to occur. However, if the condition has been present for a long time, treatment using only 'first aid' homoeopathic remedies is unlikely to be enough. In this situation, it would be wise to seek the advice of an experienced homoeopath, who will evaluate the whole person, taking into account the patient's past history and the family history.

FLUID IN THE EARS ('GLUE EAR')

Chronic catarrh. Mouth breathing. Recurrent tonsillitis.	**Kali Muriaticum 6c.** One dose morning and evening for 4–8 weeks.
Deafness – intermittently hard of hearing. Variable deafness. Squelching, bubbling noises in the ear.	**Pulsatilla 6c.** One dose morning and evening for 4–8 weeks.

If the treatment appears to cure the deafness, and your doctor finds on examination that the ear drums have returned to normal, then stop.

If however the ear drums have not completely returned to normal, or the hearing is improving but variable, continue to use the remedies for a further month and arrange for your doctor to examine the ears again.

If there is still doubt, ask to be able to consult an ENT surgeon.

SLEEPLESSNESS IN CHILDREN

This is frequently caused by overexcitement in the evening, playing too late, television, and a general lack of calm preparation for bed. Noise in the home and the neighbourhood contributes to disturbance.

Obviously, in a persisting case, all these aspects must be attended to. The child should be put to bed as tranquilly as possible. A warm drink, story-telling, a darkened room in the summer and a small night light in the winter, a warm, cosy bed with a favourite soft toy or doll, and not too much attention to the actual problem, may all help to induce sleep.

There are no homoeopathic remedies which act as sedatives, but there are several remedies which may help in particular circumstances.

SORE THROAT IN CHILDREN

See 'Sore Throat', pages 196–7.

SLEEPLESSNESS IN CHILDREN

Anxiety, restlessness. Fear and excitement.	**Aconite 30c.** One to two doses in the evening and on retiring.
Anxiety about forthcoming events (e.g. examinations) or starting a new school.	**Argentum Nitricum 6c.** One dose in the evening and on retiring.
Very restless – gets out of bed and walks about; tries to sleep in a chair or another bed. Increasingly apprehensive.	**Arsenicum Album 6c.** One to two doses in the evening and on retiring.
Nightmares. Red face, hot dry skin. Pupils dilated, eyes bright. Head hot.	**Belladonna 6c.** One to two doses in the evening and on retiring.
Oversensitive, especially to pain; peevish and petulant.	**Chamomilla 6c.** One to two doses in the evening and on retiring.
Can't stop thinking. Excitement, happy events. Very sensitive to noise.	**Coffea Cruda 6c.** One to two doses in the evening and on retiring.
Restless, miserable, depressed, afraid to be alone. Weepy and hysterical.	**Ignatia 6c.** One to two doses in the evening and on retiring.
Sensitive, mentally active, irritable and angry.	**Nux Vomica 6c.** One to two doses in the evening and on retiring.
Nightmares in a very sensitive child. Fear of the dark.	**Phosphorus 6c.** One to two doses in the evening and on retiring.

Fevers and Infectious Diseases

A high fever in a child under the age of two may result in a convulsion. This is because the brain is still immature and reacts to a high temperature in this way.

Although alarming to the observer, a febrile convulsion does not cause the child any damage. Some children are much more prone to this than others.

The first time a child has a convulsion, medical help must be sought as an emergency and the child admitted to hospital. If it is established that the convulsion was due to a high fever (febrile convulsion), the parents must be instructed to manage any future illnesses of their child rigorously. That is, as soon as the child shows signs of becoming ill, the temperature must be controlled by tepid sponging and the administration of paracetamol syrup.

The remedies on the opposite page will help to keep the temperature down, and abort the illness.

General Management

- Dress in light clothes in a warm, well-ventilated room.
  or
- Put to bed with light clothing.
- Do not overwrap or cover up the patient, or in any way raise the temperature to 'sweat it out'.
- If the temperature is raised, cool the child down by bathing it or allowing it to play with toys in the bath for longer than usual.
- Provide *and give* frequent drinks.

FEVERS AND INFECTIOUS DISEASES

First signs of onset. Dry, burning skin. Fever. Thirst, chills. Restlessness and anxiety. Worse in evening and before midnight.	**Aconite 30c**
Early stage with high fever. Dry, burning skin but wants to be covered. Red face. Dilated pupils. Swollen, tender glands.	**Belladonna 6c**
Restless and agitated. Great anxiety. Prostration. Needs warmth except to head. Hot and cold alternately. Thirsty for small amounts. Worse after midnight.	**Arsenicum Album 6c**
Very drowsy and confused. Dull-looking. Hallucinations. Temperature irregular. General bruised sensation.	**Baptisia 6c**
Shivery and sweating. Thirsty for large amounts at long intervals. Headache and pain. Worse for jarring and coughing.	**Bryonia 6c**
Low-grade fever – slow onset. Moderate thirst. Frequent sweats. Shivering, headache. Generally not much to show for the condition as a whole.	**Ferrum Phosphoricum 6c**
Heavy aching feeling of limbs and head. Drowsy. Slow onset, trembling. No thirst. Chills up and down spine.	**Gelsemium 6c**

Remember that a few doses of **Aconite 30c** at intervals of about an hour, started at the very first signs of an illness, can hasten its resolution and even abort it.

However, if the above symptoms are established give the appropriate remedy as follows: One dose every one to two hours for the first day, and reduce the frequency with improvement over the next two or three days.

CHICKENPOX

In young children, small pink spots start on the back and spread to other parts. They become fluid-filled vesicles like small glass beads or drops of water *on* the skin. Later they become yellow. The main problem is intense itching caused by the vesicles. Calamine lotion dabbed onto the skin can be very soothing. Treatment can be both of the general condition and of the skin irritation.

GLANDULAR FEVER (INFECTIOUS MONONUCLEOSIS)

This virus infection can occur in epidemics or as individual cases and affects schoolchildren, teenagers and young adults.

It starts generally as tiredness, aching muscles and headache, tender swollen glands and a fever. A sore throat which continues in spite of antibiotic treatment may arouse suspicion of glandular fever. There may be a measles-like rash in the first ten days, and later jaundice and abdominal pains.

The general picture is very vague and difficult to diagnose, and confirmation may only be possible with special blood tests.

Some patients may be ill for several weeks, with episodes of great debility, sweats and fever occurring for many months.

Treatment

The patient must be kept in bed during the times of fever and must rest at other times, and avoid any strenuous exercise.

CHICKEN POX

Prevention and contact with friends with chickenpox.	**Varicellinum 30c.** Three doses in 24 hours.
Peevish, cries easily. Hates being touched or washed. Nauseous. Very sensitive stomach.	**Antimonium Crudum 6c.** One dose three to four times a day for 4–5 days.
Pustules large. Peevish and whining. Wants company.	**Antimonium Tartaricum 6c.** One dose three to four times a day for 4–5 days.
Restless mind and body. Great itching.	**Rhus Toxicodendron 6c.** One dose three to four times a day for 4–5 days.

Continue using the remedy for two or three days after the main symptoms clear up. Ask your doctor's advice if you have any doubts about new symptoms or any worsening of the condition.

GLANDULAR FEVER (INFECTIOUS MONONUCLEOSIS)

Early Stages (see pages 96–7)

Prevention – when the child has been in contact with a confirmed case or during an outbreak at the school or in the district.	**Glandular Fever Nosode 30c.** One dose every day for 3 days, and then once a week for a month.
Weakness and debility. Headache, drowsiness. Muscular pains. Ulcerated throat, painful, difficulty swallowing. Enlarged glands. Blotchy rash.	**Ailanthus Glandulosa 6c.** One dose three times a day until improvement is maintained.

MEASLES

After starting like a common cold, the dull blotchy red rash starts behind the ears and spreads to the face, trunk and limbs. The face is puffy and the eyelids swollen. Dislike of strong light is helped by drawing curtains and using heavily shaded lights. Light will *not harm* the eyes, but only cause discomfort.

MUMPS

The severity of the illness varies from mild to severe and so does the swelling of the glands in front of the ears. Occasionally, glands under the lower jaw become swollen.

Do not give sour drinks as they may cause pain in the glands by provoking a sudden flow of saliva.

Complications are rare.

MEASLES

Prevention and contact – children not immunised and other children in the family.	**Morbillinum 30c.** Three doses in 24 hours.
Early Stage (see pages 96–7).	
Later Stage	
High temperature; chilly shivers. Dull look, swollen face, chesty. Cough causing headache.	**Bryonia 6c.** One dose three to four times a day for 4–5 days.
Running nose; watering, sore eyes. Strong light painful. Not very ill.	**Euphrasia 6c.** One dose three to four times a day for 4–5 days.
Chesty – tight feeling, dry cough. Very thirsty, wants cold water which he may vomit.	**Phosphorus 6c.** One dose three to four times a day for 4–5 days.
Restless, whingeing, wants petting and comforting. Cough troublesome. Wants cool air.	**Pulsatilla 6c.** One dose three to four times a day for 4–5 days.

MUMPS

Prevention and contact	**Parotidinum 30c.** Three doses in 24 hours.
Early Stage (see pages 96–7)	
Established Stage	
Severe headache.	**Pilocarpinum Muriaticum 3x.** One dose every two to four hours for 4–6 doses.
Afterwards.	**Pulsatilla 30c.** One dose twice a day for 3–4 days.

Pilocarpinum Muriaticum 3x will need to be ordered specially from a homoeopathic chemist.

SCARLET FEVER

This illness begins with headache, sore throat, painful neck glands and a high fever. The fine flush of a rash begins on the second day except around the mouth. This disease practically disappeared from the scene in the United Kingdom for about twenty years, but has returned with an increasing frequency in the last ten years or so. The problem here is the possibility of developing complications in the heart and kidneys, and because of this it is essential to consult your doctor at the outset. Remember to warn the doctor about any possible allergy to antibiotics.

Homoeopathic remedies are valuable when used together with your doctor's orthodox treatment. You may use the first-aid remedies on the page opposite, **but only to give you time to arrange to consult an experienced homoeopath.**

WHOOPING COUGH

See also 'Cough', pages 126–7.

This can be dangerous under the age of six months, and very troublesome under the age of one year. Starting like a cold, the harsh, dry coughs become grouped together and finally a whoop develops, with prostration and vomiting. (See 'Immunisation', overleaf.) In any event, Pertussin may be used in an attempt to prevent whooping cough and as an aid to recovery afterwards.

SCARLET FEVER

Prevention and contact during epidemics or after contacts.	**Streptococcinum 30c.** One dose every week for the duration of the epidemic.
Early Stage (see pages 96–7) Bright red face, pallor around mouth. Large pupils. Hot, dry skin. Very sore throat.	**Belladonna 6c.** One dose every two to four hours for 4–6 doses.
Profuse salivation. Sore throat and mouth, offensive breath. Chills and shivering alternating with the fever.	**Mercurius Solubilis 6c.** One dose every two to four hours for 4–6 doses.

WHOOPING COUGH

Prevention and contact during outbreaks in your district.	**Pertussin 30c.** One dose once a week for the duration of the outbreak (on medical prescription only).
Very Early Stage Dry, hard, ringing cough. Fever, thirst, hot skin. Rapid pulse. Anxiety.	**Aconite 30c.** One dose every two hours for 2–3 doses. Then proceed to one of the remedies below.
Acute Stage Barking, repetitive cough. Worse at night. Restless, crying. Hot, red, dry skin.	**Belladonna 6c.** One dose 4–6 times a day.
Fits of dry, barking cough. Worse at night. Croup (see pages 88–9).	**Drosera 6c.** One dose every 2–4 hours.
Incessant, violent cough with retching.	**Ipecacuanha 30c.** One dose 4–6 times a day.
To Follow an Attack	**Pertussin 30c.** One dose every day for 3 days (see above).

IMMUNISATION

Whilst immunisation has been of great benefit in controlling infections like diphtheria, tetanus and poliomyelitis, some children have suffered severe reactions, although a causal link has not been definitely established. All parents must decide about the use of vaccines for their own children. After taking careful advice from the doctor, the responsibility is theirs.

Children who have any of the following should either be immunised with great caution or not at all:

- Convulsions or a close family history of convulsions or epilepsy (parents or siblings).
- A bad reaction to previous immunisation.

Homoeopathic remedies made from disease products (nosodes) are used by some homoeopaths as an alternative. Although they have been used for many years and have no side effects or reactions, the degree of protection they provide has not yet been scientifically established. The policy of the UK Faculty of Homoeopathy is that all children should be conventionally immunised.

GENERAL PROBLEMS

ACNE VULGARIS
(Blackheads, Pustules, 'Blind boils')

This is a common skin condition in adolescents, caused by an imbalance in the hormone levels. It can occur later, particularly in women premenstrually, or occasionally with hormone changes during or after pregnancy or in the menopause. Some patients find that a fatty or too rich diet worsens the condition.

The spots themselves are caused by inflammation, with or without secondary infection, setting up in small sebaceous glands of the skin which have become blocked up. They may or may not be painful.

External Treatment

This should be as gentle as possible. Harsh scouring or 'strong' antiseptic soaps and ointments should be avoided. Creams and ointments containing antibiotics or the cortisone type of hormones **should not** be used, since general allergic reactions and permanent damage to the skin can easily occur.

ACNE VULGARIS
(Blackheads, Pustules, 'Blind boils')

Painful red pustules with discharging yellow pus.	**Hepar Sulphuris 6c.** One dose morning and evening.
Painful burning and stinging. *Pustules* on the face, chest, shoulder. 'Blind boils'.	**Kali Bromatum 6c.** One dose morning and evening.
Blackheads with an oily skin. Small pimples on face and forehead.	**Selenium 6c.** One dose morning and evening.

Try the most appropriate remedy listed above for three to six weeks. If only partially effective, or not effective, consult a homoeopath. Since acne is the result in the skin of a general bodily disturbance, other deeper-acting constitutional remedies may be needed.

External Treatment

Infected areas or individual spots may be helped by applying a little **Calendula** cream or ointment. If the skin is greasy, dabbing on a little of the tincture of Calendula may be better.

ANXIETY
(Anxiety state, Tension state, Feeling stressed)

Sudden short-lived anxiety due to particular circumstances is natural and needs no treatment, since after a short time the mind and body return to normal. However, with repeated episodes of acute fear and anxiety, or long-continued unrelieved anxiety, a state of 'chronic anxiety' develops. A 'chronic anxiety state' is a complex condition and does not fall within the scope of this book.

If you have been taking tranquillisers for many months or even years, you must realise that it can be **very dangerous** if such drugs are stopped suddenly. Violent reactions both physical and mental can occur. Evaluation and treatment from a homoeopathic doctor is advisable in such cases.

The homoeopathic remedies described on the opposite page differ a little from most of the others in this book because they try, very briefly, to indicate the wider aspects of the remedies and of the type of patient they are most likely to help. This, when fully developed, is called the 'constitutional approach'. It assesses the relative importance of psychological, physical, dietary, climatic and social aspects of the whole person. Generally speaking, you will not need this approach when dealing in a First Aid way with your family.

When possible, stressful situations should be avoided. When this cannot be done, one must learn, by whatever means possible, to be less affected by stress. Most people try to avoid changing any established patterns of living and thinking. Remedies alone should not be expected to compensate for the bad habits of a lifetime.

General Measures

Other measures that will help are:

- Books on self-help for your nerves.
- Tapes for relaxation.
- Courses for relaxation, e.g. yoga, meditation, breathing, autogenic training.
- Counselling.
- Avoiding stimulants, e.g. tea, coffee, nicotine.
- Regular exercise.

ANXIETY
(Anxiety state, Tension state, Feeling stressed)

(See also 'Fear', pages 136–7, and in particular the indications for **Aconite**, **Argentum Nitricum**, **Arsenicum Album** and **Gelsemium**.)

Easily anxious and discouraged. Apprehensive with palpitations. Forgetful and confused. Obstinate and slow. Flabby, chilly, dislikes activity.	**Calcarea Carbonica 30c.** One dose two to three times a day for a few days, and reduce with improvement.
Oversensitive – sighing. Problems exaggerated. Overreaction – palpitations. Insomnia, loss of appetite. Easily distracted into an improvement.	**Ignatia 30c.** One dose two to three times a day, when needed. Can be used before particular events.
Marked lack of confidence. Fears failure – covers up. Irritable and touchy. Hates contradiction.	**Lycopodium 30c.** One dose two to three times a day, and reduce with improvement.
Oversensitive. Easily fearful. Fears the dark. Needs reassurance. Restless and fidgety. Bright, emotional, loving.	**Phosphorus 30c.** One dose two to three times a day for a few days, and reduce with improvement.
Very chilly, thin and weak. Nervous, irritable, stubborn. Anxiety before events. Fears failure. Exhausted by effort.	**Silica 30c.** One dose two to three times a day, and reduce with improvement.

ARTHRITIS

There are many reasons why a joint becomes swollen and painful, from rheumatism and infection, to injury in accidents. In the latter case, you must bear in mind the general situation of the accident. All infected joints must be treated by a doctor who, after examination and investigation, will probably prescribe a suitable antibiotic. You may use the appropriate homoeopathic remedies at the same time. When joints flare up in a longstanding case of rheumatoid arthritis, you may use the homoeopathic remedies immediately.

General Measures

- Rest the joint in what, for the patient, is the most comfortable position.
- Avoid activity or weight-bearing and too much movement.
- Apply hot or cold applications, whichever give the patient the most relief of the pain, stiffness and swelling.

Homoeopathic Treatment

Note carefully when pain, stiffness and swelling are better or worse in relation to:

- The time of day or night
- The position of the affected joints
- The movement of the joints
- The stillness of the joints
- Hot or cold applications
- General weather conditions, more particular changes in the weather, e.g. hot dry, cold damp or thunder and lightning.
- If the symptom picture is right, most remedies can be used to treat both the sudden and the long-term situation.

ARTHRITIS

Sudden Onset – Acute

New Case

Very sudden onset of shiny, red hot swelling, with severe burning, stinging pains. Worse for slightest touch and pressure and local heat. Better by uncovering and cold bathing. Thirstless.	**Apis 6c** or **30c.** One dose every 10–15 minutes at first. Stop with improvement.
Bruised pain and stiffness in joints, especially in a recent injury to a long affected joint, e.g. a fall, a blow or overexertion. Worse for cold damp and slight touch.	**Arnica 6c** or **30c.** One dose every 3–4 hours. Stop with improvement.
Pains shift rapidly, usually from below upwards. Numbness and coldness in limbs. Joints swollen and hot but not red. Worse for warmth of bed and at night. Better with cold bathing.	**Ledum 6c.** One dose every 3–4 hours in an acute attack. Stop with improvement.

New Case, or a Recent Flare-up in an Old Case

Joints red, swollen and hot; very stiff with tearing and piercing pain. Worse by least movement, touch or jarring. Generally dry mouth and great thirst for large quantities of drinks. Very irritable. Generally worse in hot weather, but better with hot applications, pressure, lying on painful side and rest.	**Bryonia 6c** or **30c.** One dose every 3–4 hours. Stop with improvement.
Erratic aching or stabbing pains in swollen small joints of wrists and fingers, ankles and toes. Pains fly from joint to joint every few minutes. Can occur in any patient but is particularly useful in arthritis in menopausal women.	**Caulophyllum 6c.** One dose every 3–4 hours. Stop with improvement.

(*continued overleaf*)

ARTHRITIS (continued)

New Case, or a Recent Flare-up in an Old Case (*continued*)

Pains progress from above downwards and change position rapidly, followed by swelling. Worse with movement, and maximal about midday.

Kalmia Latifolia 6c or **30c.** One dose every 3–4 hours. One in the morning and one in the evening at a later stage. Stop with improvement.

Swollen and hot joints with muscular stiffness and tearing pain in the tissues around the joints. Better by gentle, slow movement and changes in position; by local hot applications and by hot dry weather. Worse for cold damp weather, tiredness and rest, and at the beginning of movement.

Rhus Toxicodendron 6c or **12c.** One dose every 3–4 hours. Stop with improvement.

ARTHRITIS (continued)

Chronic – Long-Term

Rheumatic pains shooting like electric shocks, shifting rapidly. Pain in ankles and feet, suddenly on and off. Restless but movement does not improve. Worse in morning and for exposure to damp cold weather. Better warmth; dry weather, rest.	**Phytolacca 6c.** One dose 3–4 times a day. Stop with improvement.
Tearing pain and swelling, worse before a storm, usually better after storm breaks and for local warmth.	**Rhododendron 6c.** One dose 3–4 times a day. Stop with improvement.
Useful in both new and old cases Joints stiff, painful, swollen, especially the big toe e.g. in gout. Very tender to slightest touch and movement. Pain flits from joint to joint. Worse for any movement, cold and at night. Better for local heat.	**Colchicum 6c** or **30c.** One dose 3–4 times a day. Stop with improvement.
Useful in older cases Dull tearing pains in deformed and swollen joints. Contractures and muscular weakness. Worse for dry, cold weather and better for warm, wet weather and warmth of bed.	**Causticum 6c** or **30c.** One dose 3–4 times a day. Stop with improvement.

CHILBLAINS AND POOR CIRCULATION

'Poor Circulation' is a loose term that explains a range of conditions from cold hands and feet, 'dead fingers', blotchy mottled legs, painful cramps and chilblains.

Chilblains can occur on the ears, the fingers and the toes. They can be described as the damage done to the tissues from a spasm of the blood vessels triggered off by the cold. An occasional episode can be treated on a first-aid basis, but recurring episodes or a lifelong problem indicate a constitutional weakness. A rather special condition called Raynaud's disease is characterised by blue or white fingers triggered by the cold, especially by placing the hands in cold water. In any of these circumstances consult an experienced homoeopath. If the condition gets worse, consult your own doctor in all cases because special investigations may be needed.

Prevention

- Stimulate the circulation by plenty of exercise.
- Hands, ears and feet should not be needlessly exposed to cold and must be protected appropriately by warm clothing and boots.
- Homoeopathic remedies can be effective in prevention. Use the remedy which may have been helpful in the previous winter. If you are new to homoeopathy use a remedy chosen on the symptoms you remember. Take one dose every week, starting at the beginning of winter, but if symptoms arise, check that you are using the right remedy and then follow the dosage on the opposite page.

CHILBLAINS AND POOR CIRCULATION

Poor Circulation

Cramps and burning pain helped by heat. Cold hands and feet.	**Arsenicum Album 6c.** One dose morning and evening. Continue for several weeks at a time.
Cramps – especially at night in old people. Coldness of hands and feet. Blotchy blue skin. Cramp of the *calves* and *feet.*	**Cuprum Metallicum 6c.** One dose morning and evening, or one dose each night on retiring.
Cold hands and feet. 'Blue' or 'dead white' fingers and toes. Pain and cramps. Burning helped by cold.	**Secale 6c.** One dose morning and evening. Continue for several weeks at a time.

Chilblains

Red swellings. Pustules. Burning, itching and prickling. Worse when cold.	**Agaricus 6c.** One dose morning and evening until relief.
Blue blotches. Stabbing pain. Worse with heat. Better for cold and exercise.	**Pulsatilla 6c.** One dose morning and evening until relief.

Tamus ointment applied twice a day to the chilblains can be very soothing.

CHRONIC FATIGUE SYNDROME

Almost every person who has had influenza, or indeed any viral infection, suffers from a period of general malaise and needs to recuperate for a time lasting from a few days to two or three weeks. Some people require longer than others, and some outbreaks of infection are noted both for their severity and the time needed for full recovery. In other words, post-viral debility, to a greater or lesser degree, is a commonplace experience.

However some patients suffer debility and sometimes more specific symptoms for a much longer time than average, up to several months or years. If the symptoms continue for more than six months, these patients can then be said to have developed what has become known as the Chronic Fatigue Syndrome (CFS) – perhaps what was called neurasthenia in Victorian times.

There is no one single cause of CFS. It is an umbrella term to cover all causes of chronic fatigue, from environmental causes such as organophosphate poisoning (e.g. from sheep-dipping), to an idiosyncratic reaction to mercury amalgam fillings, to persistent viral infections.

There is a subgroup of CFS known in the UK as myalgic encephalomyelitis (ME). This is a distinct disease entity, in which the sufferer develops perculiar, severe and variable symptoms shortly after the viral infection, and not only as a long-term development. Research has thrown light on many different aspects of ME, indicating that ME is indeed a physical disease, started by a viral infection, and not a form of depression or hysteria.

The disease commences with a severe flu-like illness and progresses into a distinctive picture with varied symptoms:

- A dreadful feeling of malaise and intense muscular weakness which is present most of the time, but which can occur with increased intensity at irregular intervals.
- Malaise made worse by physical, mental or emotional overactivity, with a far longer than usual period of recovery.
- Physical feelings of severe muscular weakness and tiredness with frustration, needing many days or even weeks to return to the previous level.
- Generalised dizziness with or without episodes of true vertigo.
- Abnormal sensations and pains, frequently with great muscular tenderness, unusual distributions, and muscular twitching and jerking.
- Unusual patterns of sweating, as well as coldness of hands and feet (Raynaud's disease), together with marked sensitivity to temperature changes and extremes.

- Altered sleeping patterns, from severe insomnia to excessive sleeping, with a reversal of diurnal rhythm.
- Confusion, loss of memory and extremely variable and labile emotions.
- Intolerance of alcohol, which lessens as improvement occurs.

Unfortunately, no specific diagnostic test for ME has yet been developed. However, homoeopathic prescribing does not depend on diagnosis, and can be based on the total symptom picture.

Even if a cure cannot be obtained, alleviation of some troublesome symptoms can be of great help to an ME patient.

General nervous excitement and incoherent talk. Manic depression, mood swings – progresses to indifference, confusion and disinclination to work. Neuralgic pains with sensation of ice-cold needles. Reading difficult, vision dim and flickering. Twitching of muscle groups. Rumbling in abdomen. Frequent urging to urinate. Irregular palpitations of heart. Stiffness and weakness of muscles. Much yawning. Burning, itching and swelling of skin.

Agaricus 6c or **30c.** One dose 2–3 times a day. Reduce with improvement.

Great debility and exhaustion after slight exertion, with nervous and physical restlessness. Worse after midnight. Great anxiety. Burning pains better with heat. Great thirst for small quantities of drink. Face pale, yellow and thin. Worse for cold weather, cold food and drinks. Better for warmth, warm food and drinks.

Arsenicum Album 6c or **30c.** One dose 2–3 times a day. Reduce with improvement.

General prostration with areas of weakness, paralysis and trembling. Dizziness, drowsiness, mental dullness. Dull headache, band-like or at back. Dusky face. Sensation of lump in throat. No thirst. Profuse, clear urine. Slow weak pulse. Bruised weak feeling in back. Cramps and trembling in all muscle groups. Double vision. Worse damp weather, excitement, bad news, before a thunderstorm. Better for motion, eventually profuse urination, fresh open air.

Gelsemium 6c or **30c.** One dose 2–3 times a day. Reduce with improvement.

CHRONIC FATIGUE SYNDROME (continued)

General muscular weakness, introspective, brooding, sad, tearful, much sighing. Changeable moods. 'Fed up', 'Had enough'. Congestive headaches. Visual disturbances. Twitching of face. Spasms of muscles. Tendency to choke with lump in throat. Spasm of rectal muscles. Headache like nail driven into side of head. Repetitive headaches. Nausea helped by eating. Better from distraction and warmth.

Ignatia 30c One dose morning and evening. Reduce with improvement.

Thin face, pale, waxy skin. Dark blotches under eyes. Physical and mental exhaustion, staggering, restless. Very chilly, vertigo and giddiness. Anxious depression, insomnia, nightmares, headaches. Fear of crowds and agoraphobia. Loss of memory, lassitude, muscular weakness, collapse. Aches and pains in limbs, worse with exercise, the cold, mental effort, sexual intercourse, crowds. Better with gentle movement, slow walking, after eating, cheerful carers.

Kali Phosphoricum 6c or **30c.** One dose 2–3 times a day. Reduce with improvement. (This remedy is probably the most used for post-influenzal symptoms.)

Sickly yellowish face with bluish-red circles around eyes. Excess salivation, moist swollen tongue. Drowsy by day, insomnia at night, nightmares. Poor memory for names, recent reading. Unable to speak clearly or calculate easily. Exhaustion after mild exertion. Vertigo with swaying. Deep muscle pains, tender bones. Stabbing and pricking pains, with alternating hot and cold sensations. Worse at night, with extremes of temperature. Better in dry warmth.

Mercurius Solubilis 6c or **30c.** One dose 2–3 times a day. Reduce with improvement.

Listless. Poor memory. Apathetic. Confusion of thinking and comprehension. Crushing headache, worse for shaking or noise. Blue rings round eyes in pale earthy face. Milky urine. Sensation of insects under skin. Aching pain in back and limbs.

Phosphoric Acid 6c or **30c.** One dose 2–3 times a day. Reduce with improvement.

Extreme muscular weakness with trembling and twitching heaviness and numbness. Legs feel as though encased in tight stockings or pricked by needles. Must lie down. Listless and indifferent to everything. No anxiety. Headaches. Vertigo on stooping, aversion to all food. Unrefreshing sleep disturbed by constant dreams. Worse from mental or physical exertion, wet weather, after sleep, stuffy atmosphere. Better lying down, cold air, sunny weather.

Picric Acid 30c. One dose every day. Reduce with improvement.

Aching weakness of limbs – feels better moving. Twitching of muscles. Nervous and forgetful, confusion and poor attention. Dull frontal headache with aching in eyeballs. Restless sleep with nightmares.

Scutellaria 6c or **30c.** One dose 2–3 times a day. Reduce with improvement.

Weakness, pallor, sunken eyes. Very chilly, staggering gait in dark. Restless legs, fine muscular twitching and trembling, can't keep feet still. Soles of feet sensitive. Numbness, coldness and abnormal sensations in arms and legs. Lethargic, depressed, irritable and oversensitive, especially to noise. Poor memory. Either increased appetite or lack of. Prolonged episodes of shivering. Sweating at night. Generally worse from alcohol.

Zincum Metallicum 6c. One dose 2–3 times a day. Reduce with improvement.

COMMON COLD – EARLY STAGES

Colds and influenza are infectious illnesses caused by viruses. There are many types and they vary from year to year.

The resistance of the individual to these viruses is of great importance and this depends on good general health. General health, in its turn, depends upon high quality nourishing foods, adequate rest and recreation, the absence of prolonged or severe stress and daily physical exercise. A deficiency of any of these can weaken the health as a whole, and the person becomes prone to illness.

Homoeopathic treatment can be used to improve the resistance to infection. Well selected remedies will speed up the cure and reduce the development of catarrh, sinusitis and bronchitis.

See also the discussions in the section on 'Fevers and Infectious Diseases', pages 96–103; 'Cough', pages 126–7; 'Influenza', pages 158–9; and 'Sore Throat', pages 196–7.

General Management

- Go home and stay away from other people, if possible. This is important during the first day or so, when you are very infectious.
- Take extra vitamin C – up to 500mg twice a day – especially if you have a temperature.
- Choose a remedy from the list opposite and change it if the symptoms change. If you cannot decide which is the better of two remedies take them alternately at intervals of one hour.

COMMON COLD – EARLY STAGES

Prevention	**'Cold and Flu tablets'.** One tablet morning and evening on the first (and perhaps also the 15th) day of each month.

Early Stages

Very first signs of a cold. Sudden chill, shivering. Fever.	**Aconite 30c.** One dose every 2 hours, for the first day – into the second day or overnight.
Very sore raw nostrils and upper lip caused by profusely running nose. Sneezing. Painless watery eyes.	**Allium Cepa 6c.** One dose every 2 hours until improvement, and then reduce.
Stiff neck and pain in the throat, back and limbs. Eyes and nose streaming. Sneezing. Brought on by being chilled when hot, or drenched in cold wet weather.	**Dulcamara 6c.** One dose every 2 hours until improvement, and then reduce.
Eyes red and sore from burning tears. Profuse watery nasal discharge. Sneezing.	**Euphrasia 6c.** One dose every 2 hours until improvement, and then reduce.
Cold starting with sneezing. Patient chilly and introverted.	**Natrum Muriaticum 6c.** One dose every 2 hours until improvement, and then reduce.
Sudden intense chill with shivering. Unable to get warm. Patient irritable. Nose dry and stuffed up.	**Nux Vomica 6c.** One dose every 2 hours until improvement, and then reduce.

If the chosen remedy does not relieve your symptoms within twenty-four hours it is probable that it is not the correct one. Reassess the symptoms at this stage and make a further choice.

COMMON COLD – LATER STAGES

As a rule people tend to follow their own patterns in the way that a cold develops. Occasionally a particular type of infection will impose its own pattern on the patient.

From the homoeopathic point of view this does not matter – you choose the remedy by matching the main symptoms of the patient and the remedy.

The tendency is for the watery discharge of the early cold to become secondarily infected. Yellow or green catarrh develops at this point, and can be thick and difficult to dislodge. The infection may spread to the chest or to the throat or ears.

General Management

- Avoid overexposure to bad weather and avoid other people with infections.
- Take it easy for a few days – give the body a chance to throw off the whole illness.
- Use steam inhalations to help the catarrh to disperse, but do not use strong-smelling substances such as vapour rubs or Oil of Eucalyptus or Friar's Balsam. These may antidote the effects of the homoeopathic remedies you are taking.
- Continue to change the remedies as the symptoms change.

COMMON COLD – LATER STAGES

'Flu-like cold'. Heavy head, tired heavy eyes. Backache with shivers up and down. Arms and legs ache. Sore nose. Wants to lie down and sleep.	**Gelsemium 6c.** One dose at intervals of 1–2 hours and reduce with improvement.
Stringy, yellow nasal discharge, sticky and difficult to shift. Post-nasal drip.	**Hydrastis 6c.** One dose at intervals of 1–2 hours and reduce with improvement.
Thick, sticky, yellow or green nasal discharge. May be bloodstained, difficult to blow out. Thick, sticky crusts in nose.	**Kali Bichromicum 6c.** One dose at intervals of 1–2 hours and reduce with improvement.
Pain over the eyes. Stinging, watery nasal discharge. Violent sneezing. Smarting, watering eyes.	**Kali Iodatum 6c.** One dose at intervals of 1–2 hours and reduce with improvement.
Thick, yellow, burning nasal discharge. Nostrils may be raw and ulcerated. Profuse sweating or chilled and shivering even in a hot room. Offensive breath.	**Mercurius Solubilis 6c.** One dose at intervals of 1–2 hours and reduce with improvement.
Thick, greenish-yellow catarrh. Stuffy nose at night and indoors. Generally better in fresh air.	**Pulsatilla 6c.** One dose at intervals of 1–2 hours and reduce with improvement.

CONSTIPATION

A person is constipated when he or she repeatedly fails to have a regular bowel action. The motion may be large and bulky, either soft or hard, but it may also be small lumps more or less crammed together. The basic fact is that the bowel is not cleared on a regular basis.

Many people become constipated because they never develop the habit of going to the toilet as soon as they feel the urge to move their bowels. In this way 'the urge' gradually becomes weaker – and the bowels are moved less frequently and eventually the retention of bowel contents results.

It is a mistake to resort to laxatives, and prevention is better than cure.

You must consult your doctor if the constipation has been getting worse over several weeks or months, or if you have used laxatives regularly and now find that you need more to achieve the same result.

You should also consult your doctor if the constipated motion is passed with blood or mucus, or if piles develop and increase in severity.

General Management

- Increase the amount of fibre in the diet. This is best done by eating wholemeal bread and cereals and by increasing the quantity of fruit and vegetables eaten daily. At the same time, eliminate highly-refined and manufactured foods; in short, cut out 'junk food' and eat a wholefood diet.
- Drink more liquids throughout the day. You should aim at about three pints of liquid of one sort or another in twenty-four hours. Obviously, you should drink more if you perspire profusely because of hot weather or hard exercise.
- Establish a regular time to go to the toilet.
- Use the appropriate remedy on the opposite page . If there is doubt about the most suitable remedy, take **Nux Vomica 6c** each evening and **Sulphur 6c** each morning for several days.

CONSTIPATION

Soft, sticky, unformed stool. No urge to use the bowels. Loss of expulsive power. Straining with great effort.	**Alumina 6c.** One dose morning and evening until improvement.
Small, variable stools. Frequent, ineffective urging with feeling of incomplete emptying. Lack of regular bowel habits. Over-use of laxatives in the past.	**Nux Vomica 6c.** One dose morning and evening until improvement.
Stools of small, hard, dry balls which may be packed together. No urge to use the bowels. Poor appetite.	**Opium 6c.** One dose morning and evening until improvement.
Stools large, hard and difficult to expel – they seem to slip back. Spasm of muscles of the anus. Worse during menstrual periods.	**Silica 6c.** One dose morning and evening until improvement.
Small, hard, dry stools. Great effort with pain and burning. Constipation may alternate with diarrhoea.	**Sulphur 6c.** One dose morning and evening until improvement.

COUGH

Coughing is due to irritation in the respiratory tract at any point between the larynx (voice box) and the deeper parts of the lungs.

A cough may flare up suddenly, caused by dust, fumes or smoke. Usually it occurs as part of an overall picture of a throat or chest infection. The chest infection may have developed from a cold or it may have started 'on the chest'.

However, for the purposes of a book such as this, coughs can be divided into three main groups, (although there is likely to be an overlapping of symptoms). These are:

- Dry, hacking coughs – e.g. laryngitis.
- Spasmodic, repetitive coughs – e.g. whooping cough.
- Loose coughs, with phlegm or sputum – e.g. bronchitis.

General Management

The patient should avoid places where the cough is worsened, such as dusty or smoky places, or very cold, damp weather outside. If the general condition is not improving, he or she should stay indoors, or even go to bed, or use inhalations of steam. The latter must be carefully supervised, to prevent scalding.

Call the doctor if:

- The overall condition worsens.
- There are other problems, such as diabetes or a heart condition.
- The new infection is in addition to a long-term chest infection such as chronic bronchitis or emphysema.

Do not attempt to treat severe bronchitis or pneumonia yourself. The doctor may have to prescribe an antibiotic, which at some stage could be in the best interest of the patient.

If you cannot decide which of two remedies is the more appropriate in the circumstances, take them alternately, as often as is necessary for relief. Remember to change the remedy with a change in the symptom picture.

Dry Cough

Croup-like cough in very dry, cold weather. Anxiety and restlessness. Fever, thirst, no sweating.	**Aconite 30c.** One dose at fifteen minute intervals, reducing with improvement.

COUGH

Slow, gradual fever; irritation of air passages. Cough worse for movement and entering a warm room; can be worse at night. Much thirst for cold drinks. Stabbing pains in throat or chest.

Bryonia 6c. One dose at fifteen minute intervals, reducing with improvement.

Rough, noisy croup-like cough. Sudden onset in cold weather. Better in a warm, steamy room.

Hepar Sulphuris 6c. One dose at fifteen minute intervals, reducing with improvement.

Raw, tearing, burning pain in a croup-like cough. Improves with hot drinks.

Spongia 6c. One dose at fifteen minute intervals, reducing with improvement.

Spasmodic Cough

Crowing spasmodic cough. Better for sipping cold water.

Cuprum Metallicum 6c. One dose at 15 minute intervals, reducing with improvement.

Dry cough – a bit like whooping cough. Worse at night and lying down. May be wheezing; occasionally croup- like.

Drosera 6c. One dose at 15 minute intervals, reducing with improvement.

Spasms of coughing; the more he coughs, the more he has to.

Ignatia 6c. One dose morning and evening and after a bout of coughing.

Loose Cough

Loose phlegm, thick and difficult to cough up. Breathless. Wheezing, noisy chest.

Antimonium Tartaricum 6c. One dose 4–6 times a day, reducing with improvement.

Spasmodic cough, worse in open air. Breathless. Rapid development of phlegm which may be vomited up.

Ipecacuanha 6c. One dose 4–6 times a day, reducing with improvement.

Thick yellow loose phlegm. Runny nose. Cough productive in day and dry at night. Better in fresh air. Towards end of illness.

Pulsatilla 6c. One dose 4–6 times a day, reducing with improvement.

CYSTITIS

This is a condition of the bladder which causes painful urination, with frequency during the day and often disturbed nights. There may also be incontinence, urgency and very painful bladder spasms.

Cystitis is usually caused by infection and can be treated homoeopathically very successfully although in some cases antibiotic treatment may be necessary. If this happens, homoeopathic remedies can be used as well, and the need for prolonged antibiotic treatment may be reduced or eliminated.

Caution

There are other causes for these symptoms. The patient with more than one episode of acute cystitis **must** consult the family doctor, with a view to full investigation of the urinary tract as a whole. Provided that serious disease has been excluded by the appropriate medical tests, homoeopathic medicine may be more beneficial than some orthodox medical treatments.

General Advice

- Empty bladder after sexual intercourse.
- Increase fluid intake to 1½ litres per day.
- Avoid tea, coffee and alcohol.

CYSTITIS

Stinging, burning pain before, during and after urinating. Very frequent. Small quantities of dark urine with or without blood.

Cantharis 6c. One dose at intervals of thirty minutes to one hour – reduce with improvement.

Frequency, leaking. Dribbling. Difficulty in starting. Incontinence.

Causticum 30c. One dose 2–3 times a day.

Frequency with much urine. Pain *during* and *after* completion. Bladder feels weary between urination. Bed wetting in children.

Equisetum 6c. One dose 3–4 times a day – reduce with improvement.

Frequency, urgency. Very painful spasms of bladder. Burning pain with little or no urine. Dark bloody urine.

Mercurius Corrosivus 6c. One dose at intervals of thirty minutes to one hour – reduce with improvement.

Frequency, unbearable pain at end. Urination easier standing. Urine scanty, deposits blood.

Sarsaparilla 6c. One dose at intervals of thirty minutes to one hour – reduce with improvement.

'Honeymoon cystitis' in women. Burning pains in the urethra, especially between urinating. Pain better passing urine.

Staphysagria 6c. One dose twice a day for one week.

Staphysagria can be used on a regular basis for women who suffer urethritis/cystitis each time after intercourse. Take three times a week, or following intercourse. If problems persist, consult an experienced homoeopath.

DENTAL ABSCESS (GUM BOILS)

In this condition an abscess has formed at some point around a tooth; that is, pus is forming a 'gum boil'. A dentist must be consulted and will probably prescribe an antibiotic before operating to drain the abscess.

Before this, the most suitable homoeopathic remedy on the opposite page will greatly help the condition. It can be used together with an antibiotic, if prescribed.

After the dental procedure, the dentist may advise hot salt mouth washes as frequently as possible. This is a good initial cleansing procedure, but it is only necessary to do this two or three times. Afterwards, use a mouth wash made up of 5–10 drops of **Calendula** or **Hypercal** tincture in a glass of cool, previously boiled water.

DENTAL ABSCESS (GUM BOILS)

Any of the remedies listed on page 199 for toothache may be helpful. The following remedies may also be of value.

Oral Treatment

Rubbed over the swelling as frequently as needed.	**Hypericum tincture** or **Hypercal tincture:** every 2–3 hours. Stop with improvement.

By Mouth

Throbbing, hot, shining, swelling. May have malaise and headache. Usually before pus is obvious.	**Belladonna 6c.** One dose every hour. Stop with improvement.
Early swelling, but pus not ready to discharge. To speed up abscess formation.	**Hepar Sulphuris 6c.** One dose every hour. Stop with improvement.
Pus discharging. Unwell. Foul taste.	**Pyrogen 6c.** One dose every hour. Stop with improvement.

DIARRHOEA

Sudden Onset

This term refers to the passing of very loose or watery motions which may contain blood, slime or, on occasion, pieces of undigested food, and which may smell offensive. Usually it is caused by infection from food or water, or by overeating fruit or unusual foods. All of these can occur on holiday in hot sunny countries.

The homoeopathic remedies on the opposite page should prove helpful for these situations. For the traveller and holiday maker, **Arsenicum Album** (or failing that, **Veratrum Album**) will probably be the most usual remedies. If the diarrhoea persists, then one of the other remedies listed might be more appropriate. Antibiotics are not helpful in general, and too often bring about a reactive diarrhoea and other complications.

In very hot weather, old people and children can dehydrate rapidly. This must be prevented by giving frequent drinks.

In nervous adults and in children, diarrhoea can arise from fears and anxiety. Here the answer is to treat the person as a whole in relation to the type of anxiety. (See also 'Anxiety', pages 108–9 and 'Fear', pages 136–7.)

Caution

If the acute bouts and pains of diarrhoea recur at intervals of weeks or months, or if there is blood or slime in the motions, or if the patient loses weight and is generally unwell, it is **essential** that you consult your doctor for further investigation.

DIARRHOEA

Sudden Onset

Severe watery, burning and stinging diarrhoea. Chill, weakness, anxiety or prostration. Usually vomiting, but thirsty for small drinks. Can be worse after midnight. Food poisoning. Travellers' diarrhoea. Contaminated water.

Arsenicum Album 6c. One dose every two to three hours and reduce with improvement, or one dose after each motion.

Great weakness and vomiting. Bitter taste, hungry with no appetite. Painful, windy rumbling; distension. Diarrhoea with wind, worse after fruit and milk.

China 6c. One dose every two to three hours and reduce with improvement, or one dose after each motion.

Painful cramps, which start and finish suddenly. Improvement by bending double, by heat and by strong pressure.

Colocynthis 6c. One dose every two to three hours and reduce with improvement, or one dose after each motion.

Great nausea not helped by vomiting. Motion smelly, frothy, yellow or green. Colicky pain and straining. Diarrhoea in spasms. No thirst, clean tongue.

Ipecacuanha 6c. One dose every two to three hours and reduce with improvement, or one dose after each motion.

Severe, gushing watery diarrhoea; rumbling of wind; ill-smelling. Worse in morning. Colicky pains beforehand; urging afterwards. Weak feeling afterwards. Pain improved by heat and by lying on abdomen.

Podophyllum 6c. One dose every two to three hours and reduce with improvement, or one dose after each motion.

Morning diarrhoea – drives patient out of bed. Warm-blooded. Craves sweets and fats.

Sulphur 6c. One dose morning and night until improvement.

ECZEMA

This is the name given to many different conditions of the skin, from dry flaking to moist, oozing and sometimes cracking and bleeding skin. The affected area of skin frequently itches severely. This can cause distressing loss of sleep, with irritability and loss of efficiency at work or school. Scratching can introduce infections with further complications, and if continued over a long time can cause an unhealthy thickening of the skin.

The cause of eczema is a breakdown in the defence mechanisms of the body resulting in an allergic or sensitivity reaction. There can be great variation in how long the condition lasts. Stress may cause it to flare up.

Babies developing 'infantile eczema' may have been allergic to cows' milk protein in bottle feeds or to 'foreign' protein in immunisation injections. Usually there will be relations within the family who have allergic conditions like asthma, hay fever, 'dermatitis', or very specific allergies to certain foods or chemicals in make-up or detergents.

The remedies given on the page opposite are intended for First Aid only. It is essential that long-term treatment should only be undertaken by an experienced homoeopath.

External Treatment

Avoid using applications containing antibiotics and cortisone-type drugs as much as possible. However, in severe situations, remember that medical advice must be taken and corticosteroid preparations may in fact be lifesaving.

Dry eczema may be helped better by applying soothing, bland cream or ointment, for example, **Urtica Urens** cream, depending upon the patient's individual response. Frequent moisturising is very important part of eczema treatment.

Weeping and infected eczemas are probably best treated by **Calendula** lotion. Using freshly prepared lotion 5ml (20 drops) in 200ml (half a pint) of cool, previously boiled water, moisten (and keep moist) with applications of sterile gauze squares. These should be changed less frequently as the condition improves. Occasionally **Graphites** ointment can be helpful.

Itching may be helped by **Paeonia** ointment or **Urtica Urens** ointment.

ECZEMA

Dry Eczema

Unwashed, grey, greasy skin. Eczema at bends of knees and elbows. Irritation worse with cold. Patient chilly also.

Psorinum 6c. One dose morning and evening. Stop with improvement.

Dry red itching areas, especially on hands, wrists and in the bends of joints. Generally eased by warmth and much worse in cold, damp weather. Small blisters.

Rhus Toxicodendron 6c. One dose a day for a week and then one dose morning and evening until improvement is maintained.

Hot, sweaty patient with rough itching skin. Some patches of infection. Irritation worse with washing and heat of the bed.

Sulphur 6c. One dose on alternate days for a week and then one every day. Note: *Stop* if there is a reaction, wait for it to settle and then recommence treatment.

Moist Eczema

Oozing, clear or yellow discharge; 'honey-like'. Any area, but common behind ears and on the head.

Graphites 6c. One dose morning and evening.

Continue the treatment until an improvement is established, and then stop. If the eczema seems to be starting again, start the treatment again.

FEAR

See also 'Anxiety', pages 108–9.

Fear is a serious symptom and is usually an obvious response to an obvious cause. In certain cases no cause is obvious. Sometimes the fear is not simply a sudden reaction, but a recurring one when presented with the same situation. It is then known as a 'phobic anxiety state', e.g. claustrophobia or agoraphobia. In other cases the fear seems like a continuous state of heightened anxiety.

The homoeopathic remedies on the page opposite will, if chosen correctly, help in the management of the condition; other measures, such as psychotherapy, may also be required. Certainly, a long-established problem will have to be very carefully assessed by a homoeopath before starting treatment. Treatment may take months to be effective.

With minor difficulties, such as stage fright or examination nerves, the remedy can be given on going to bed for a few nights before the event, and on the morning or afternoon of the event itself.

You will notice that the potencies suggested are higher than usual. Use the 30c potency first, and if this is not entirely successful ask your chemist to get the 200c potency for you. In case of difficulty, any of the organisations listed on pages 216–17 can give you the addresses of homoeopathic chemists who supply by post.

FEAR

Sudden panic, terror or shock. Can be 'out of the blue'. Agitated, nightmares. Can over-breathe and produce palpitations and numbness, or tingling sensations in the cheeks, hands or feet.	**Aconite 30c** or **200c.** One dose immediately and repeat at fifteen minute intervals as necessary.
Apprehension before an event; 'Exam nerves' or 'stage fright'. Panic in a crowd, lift, tube station. Agitated. Patient moves rapidly.	**Argentum Nitricum 30c** or **200c.** One dose before the event if possible or repeat as necessary.
Give after acute shocks or accidents	**Arnica 30c** or **200c.** One dose immediately and repeat every half hour as necessary.
Dread – unaccountable fear. Physical and mental restlessness. Fears being alone, especially late at night. Chilly.	**Arsenicum Album 30c** or **200c.** One dose immediately and repeat every half hour as necessary.
Trembling weakness, 'paralysed by fear'. 'All of a dither'. Mind blank, can't speak or think. 'Exam nerves', 'stage fright'.	**Gelsemium 30c** or **200c.** One dose before the event if possible or repeat as necessary.
Persisting fear. Fear returning after remembering the fear-inducing event.	**Opium 30c** or **200c.** One dose at the time and repeat every day for 3–4 days.

FIBROSITIS (MUSCULAR RHEUMATISM)

This is a painful condition of the long muscles of the limbs and back. There may be sore and aching pains, spasmodic shooting pains or a sensitivity and tenderness, either generally in the whole muscle or in small swollen parts of the muscle (rheumatic nodules). The precise definition of fibrositis has been much debated over the years, and fashion plays a great part in what is meant by it. Most people with painful muscles know what they mean by it, and it is to them that this section is directed.

Local treatments are found to be very helpful in allaying the pain and stiffness and these include:

- Massage – with or without embrocations and oils.
- Local heat – electric heating pads, or diathermy, or hot water bathing (rarely, cold applications or sprays are of more help).
- Gentle passive movement.

General Treatment

Use whatever of the above methods of active treatment you have available to ease the pain and discomfort.

Observe the conditions at the start of pains and discomfort, e.g. icy cold winds after strenuous exercise with much sweating; or a chill after getting soaking wet in cold wet weather.

Observe also the general conditions which affect the pains and discomfort, e.g. cold damp or hot dry weather; gentle or vigorous exercise; hot or cold applications; keeping still or moving about; gentle or firm pressure to the affected area.

Homoeopathic Treatment

Make a careful note of all the things which ease or worsen the pains and discomfort and use them to choose one of the homoeopathic remedies on the page opposite. Also refer to:

- 'Arthritis', pages 110–13.
- The appropriate section on pains in general, pages 172–9.

FIBROSITIS (MUSCULAR RHEUMATISM)

Severe, sudden pains, brought on by cold draughts. Sudden high temperature – frequently starting with shivering; skin red and dry, no perspiration. Intense anxiety.

Aconite 6c. One dose every 4 hours. Stop with improvement.

Sore, bruised feeling, aches, pains and stiffness; impression that the bed is too hard. Present condition may have been caused by injury. Worse for touch, movement, damp cold. Better on rising.

Arnica 6c or **30c.** One dose 3–4 times a day. Stop with improvement.

Aching, stitching, tearing pain. Worse for any movement, hot weather, touch. Better for rest, pressure and keeping still, lying on painful part, local heat only.

Bryonia 6c. One dose 3–4 times a day. Stop with improvement.

Tearing, shooting pains in limbs. Brought on or made worse by cold damp conditions, or cold wet weather. Rheumatic pains alternate with indigestion or skin problems. Better for warmth, dry weather and movement.

Dulcamara 6c. One dose 3–4 times a day. Stop with improvement.

Pains worse at night and in damp weather, when lying on affected parts, and in warm rooms. Better for movement and open air.

Kali Iodatum 6c. One dose 3–4 times a day. Stop with improvement.

Tearing pains with stiffness and rigidity. Worse for cold damp weather and after rain; resting. Better for warm dry weather, slow movement, changes of position and local warmth. Pain initially worse with movement; improves when movement is continued and reappears when overdone.

Rhus Toxicodendron 6c or **30c.** One dose 3–4 times a day. Stop with improvement.

Ligaments tender. Stiffness and general aching. Worse after effort, cold wet conditions, lying down. Better for movement – like Rhus Toxicodendron.

Ruta 6c or **30c.** One dose 3–4 times a day. Stop with improvement.

HANGOVER (ILL EFFECTS OF ALCOHOL)

There can be few adults who have not had at least one episode of feeling nauseously unwell after drinking one or other of the multitude of alcoholic drinks. Usually it is by drinking too much that the troubles arise, but some people find that a particular type of drink (e.g. beer, whisky or red wine) is the cause. Occasionally the problems are caused by drinking a succession of alcoholic drinks from different sources (e.g. beer followed by wine or spirits).

Rarely, there are people who have a great sensitivity to alcohol so that even one drink brings on a whole adverse reaction, and occasionally a migraine picture.

Reactions consist of various headaches, nausea and vomiting, diarrhoea, malaise with generalised aches and pains, drowsiness or insomnia and mental confusion and lack of concentration.

Alcohol by itself can do all of these things, but the blame for a hangover lies also with the various chemicals added to most drinks.

Avoiding a Hangover

- Do not drink to excess.
- Avoid drinks which you know will cause you trouble later.
- Take food at the same time.
- Drink lots of water before going to bed.

Extra Precautions

- Do not drive or handle machinery after drinking alcohol.
- Be aware that you may not be mentally or physically functioning normally for up to twelve or twenty-four hours after drinking heavily.

Dosage

Take the first dose of the appropriate remedy with the onset of the symptoms, and repeat every ten to thirty minutes until there is improvement, and then reduce the frequency of dosage.

If the symptoms change, reassess them and if necessary give a different remedy. Once you discover which particular remedy helps you, it may be given before the actual onset of the symptoms, e.g. on retiring to bed.

HANGOVER (ILL EFFECTS OF ALCOHOL)

Anxious, very impatient and agitated. Pains in head, throbbing and shooting, very sensitive to noise, light and conversation. Pain in eyes with bright light. Cold sweating. Nausea and vomiting. Generally better for warmth and local heat.	**Arsenicum Album 30c**
Great weakness. Throbbing headache, buzzing in ears, dizziness, better for warmth and pressure. Apathetic and depressed. Hypersensitive to noise, light, touch and taste. Cannot do mental work.	**China 30c**
Heavy, congestive headache with heavy feeling, especially in the back, from the base of the skull down the neck and across the shoulders. Pain in eyeballs with heaviness of eyelids and a drowsy look; occasionally double vision, improved by sitting up and eventually by passing a large quantity of urine. Worse lying flat or with head low.	**Gelsemium 30c**
Thin, dark, tense person. Nervous and quarrelsome. Very easily offended. Sensitive to noise and light. General sore, bruised, thick head, with more marked pain over the back of the head or over one of the eyes. Generally worse from cold draughts or getting up in morning, or mental effort. Better from warmth and holding head firmly.	**Nux Vomica 30c**
Deep sleep, loud snoring, mouth open, with dry mouth and tongue. Nausea. Congestion of head with red face. Confusion and stupidity. Hot perspiration, feels too hot in bed – looks for a cool place. Slow pulse and slow noisy breathing.	**Opium 30c**

HAY FEVER

This seems to be an increasingly common condition during the summer. It is due to a sensitivity or allergy to the pollens of trees, shrubs, flowers and grasses and, occasionally, to the spores of fungi. Generally the problem is limited to one part of the season, but sometimes it may spread from spring through the summer and on to the autumn.

The symptoms may vary from year to year, may or may not be affected by the weather or the pollen count, and may get steadily worse, or fade away.

The usual picture of hay fever is one of sneezing with either a blocked or runny nose, red, itching and watering eyes, or itching at the back of the nose or throat or in the ears. There may occasionally be a tightness of the chest or even asthma, and more rarely still, an actual fever.

The treatment of the underlying cause of the sensitivity may be very complex and needs the help of a homoeopath if the cure is to be permanent.

The remedies on the page opposite are a few of the most helpful ones which can be used as first aid. If you are not able to choose a remedy accurately, or if your choice is not effective, alternate the two remedies which seem to be nearest to the symptoms of the patient.

HAY FEVER

Bouts of sneezing. Burning, watery nasal discharge. Sore nostrils and upper lip. Eyes itching, painless watering. Tickling cough.	**Allium Cepa 6c.** One dose 2–4 times a day. Reduce with improvement.
Loss of sense of smell. Nose itching, stuffy and obstructed and unable to clear by blowing. Nostrils and upper lip sore.	**Ammonium Muriaticum 6c.** One dose 2–4 times a day. Reduce with improvement.
Itching eyes. Itching roof of mouth and back of throat. Itching deep in the ears. Itching nostrils. Sneezing – loss of smell.	**Arundo 6c.** One dose 2–4 times a day. Reduce with improvement.
Sneezing, watery nose (but not sore). Eyes red, burning tears, swollen lids. Dislikes bright light. General headache.	**Euphrasia 6c.** One dose 2–4 times a day. Reduce with improvement.
Sneezing (violent). Cough. Nose running, or burning and dry. Eyes hot. Heavy, swollen eyelids. Throat tingling, dry and burning. Face flushed and heavy-looking.	**Gelsemium 6c.** One dose 2–4 times a day. Reduce with improvement.
Bouts of sneezing. Profuse, watery nasal discharge. Numbness and itching of the throat (the patient tries to scratch it with the back of the tongue). Very sensitive to strong scents. Sinus pains over the eyes. Sensation of lump in throat – needs to swallow.	**Sabadilla 6c.** One dose 2–4 times a day. Reduce with improvement.

One method of treating hay fever is to take one tablet of **Mixed Pollen 30c** each day. Many patients find that this remedy clears up the symptoms completely, while most find them much reduced. However, there are some patients whose improvement only begins when they stop taking the remedy, having taken it for a week or two. The improvement may last for several weeks.

The remedy **Grass 30c** may be a help to those people who are affected by mowing the lawn. One tablet may be taken before and after mowing.

HEADACHE AND MIGRAINE

Seek medical advice as soon as possible if the patient has a headache:

- with a stiff neck and a high fever.
- after a head injury (see pages 20–1).
- which becomes more frequent or constant.
- starting after taking prescribed medicines, especially birth control pills.

Causes of Headaches and Migraines

- Family tendency.
- Long continued stress with inadequate adaptation or inability to relax and recover from the stress.
- Food allergies or sensitivities, e.g. sweets and chocolate, coffee, fruit and nuts.
- Going without food, e.g. missing meals on journeys.
- Sleeping too long, particularly at the weekends.
- Relaxing after a stress has ended, e.g. *after* examinations in students, or at the end of a business crisis, or at the end of a stressful working week – the 'weekend headache'.
- Bright sunshine; strong flickering lights, e.g. at discos or badly adjusted TV sets or computer screens.
- Overindulgence in foods, alcohol, coffee or tobacco.

A migraine is not simply a severe headache but a generalised illness and head pain, sometimes mainly one-sided, and is only a part of the symptom picture. This recurs at certain times of the week or month or in groups at much longer intervals (*cluster headaches*).

In women these recurring patterns of headaches can occur in the middle of the menstrual cycle (i.e. ovulation time) or before, during, or after the menstrual period itself. They may also occur in girls at puberty when the menstrual period is establishing itself, or in older women when menstruation is ceasing.

Migraine headaches particularly may have additional features:

- The day before the attack the patient may be abnormally tired or feel unusually well.
- There may be diarrhoea before the attack, or nausea and vomiting during it, in some cases preceded by a profuse flow of unusual tasting saliva.
- In addition to the general throbbing or congestive pain there may be neuralgic pains in the head, eyes, neck, face and teeth.

- There may be dizziness or actual vertigo.
- There may be flashing lights or partial loss of vision.
- During the episode the patient may sweat profusely, with or without a fever.
- A very large quantity of urine may be passed and in some patients this heralds the end of the headache.

Non-Medical Treatment

- Attention to lifestyle, making time for regular exercise, not overworking, and taking holidays at intervals.
- Avoiding items of diet which are known to cause headaches, e.g. alcohol, certain cheeses, oranges, nuts, chocolates, sweets and strong coffee.
- Adequate relaxation, including special techniques such as yoga, transcendental meditation, autogenic training and simple physical relaxation as taught by physiotherapists.
- Massage for habitual muscle tension in the neck and shoulders.
- Just taking time off work.

Sudden Onset – Acute

Onset with exposure to severe heat or cold or as a result of fear, excitement or emotional crisis. Severe bursting, burning, throbbing or tearing pains. Congestion of head and face. Worse for light, heat, motion or noise. Becomes anxious, fearful and restless with the pain.	**Aconite 30c.** One dose every 15–30 minutes. Stop with improvement.
Onset in morning as a severe stabbing pain through the head, together with general congestion, brought on by stopping of some discharge, e.g. catarrh or menstruation or emotional stress. Flushed congested face, dilated pupils and bright looking eyes. Very much worse from heat and movement. Very excited, irritable and hates being disturbed. Better for firm pressure and cold applications, but tender scalp.	**Apis 30c.** One dose every 15–30 minutes. Stop with improvement.

(continued overleaf)

HEADACHE AND MIGRAINE (continued)

Starts with emotional stress or the stopping of a discharge, or exposure to heat – especially the sun – or to severe cold, after a haircut or washing one's hair. Usually starts late afternoon and continues through the night. Hot, dry head. Very bright red flushed face, without perspiration. Worse for light, motion, stooping, and movement of eyes. Pulsating pain, better for firm pressure. Patient feels chilly – better covering up. Better propped up and head held back.	**Belladonna 30c.** One dose every 15–30 minutes. Stop with improvement.
Starts during night, but only becomes aware of it after waking and moving about. Dull, deep aching in forehead – spreads through head to the back. Feeling of heaviness and heat. Generally feels chilly – cold hands and feet. Using eyes causes pain. Even hair is sensitive to touch, but better by firm pressure, and lying still and cold applications. Worse for motion or jarring. Irritable. Dislikes talking.	**Bryonia 30c.** One dose every 15–30 minutes. Stop with improvement.
Starts after a long journey or strain of night-nursing for several nights, or students after very little sleep before examinations. Very tired, exhausted and may be giddy. Curious alternate sensation of head feeling empty and numb followed by bursting pain with nausea and possibly vomiting. Worse at back of head – tenderness. Worse for short sleep, coffee, alcohol and particularly tobacco, sudden motion, mental effort. Dislikes hot rooms. Better in cold air.	**Cocculus 30c.** One dose every 15–30 minutes. Stop with improvement.

Patient looks like he is suffering from sunstroke or heat stroke. Dusky purple, puffy congestion of face. Skin moist. Pain bursting. Worse effort, straining or motion. Temporary loss of sight, or flashes of light. Better for keeping very still and ice cold applications, or gripping head in hands. May occasionally be one-sided, with flushing and dilated blood vessels on that side. Pain usually starts at sunrise, is worse at midday and gets better at sunset.	**Glonoinum 30c.** One dose every 15–30 minutes. Stop with improvement.
After emotional crisis – great disappointment or grief in a very sensitive, emotionally volatile patient. After much weeping. Sometimes feels hungry with pain; food initially relieves but later is much worse. Congestion in forehead; may also have spasmodic pains in a very small area of the head. Nausea. Worse for coffee, tobacco and alcohol. Better for being quiet, still, and by pressure. Worse for noise, light or movement and further emotional disturbance.	**Ignatia 30c**. One dose every 15–30 minutes. Stop with improvement.
Sudden onset from exposure to cold or cold winds. Neuralgic shooting pains in the head. Pallor. Very sensitive to light touch, but better for firm pressure and warmth. Worse for cold draughts.	**Magnesium Phosphoricum 30c**. One dose every 15–30 minutes. Stop with improvement.

(*continued overleaf*)

HEADACHE AND MIGRAINE (continued)

See 'Hangover' (pages 140–1). Overdrinking and overeating the night before, or staying up too late and missing sleep. Congestion over whole head, with pressure in the forehead to the top of the head. Usually constipated. Nausea and vomiting may not be present. Usually worse on waking. Bad tempered, irritable and chilly. Worse for moving or being disturbed; mental activity; taking food, alcohol or coffee. Better for lying down and wrapping up head, in a warm room; and eventually from getting up and about. Suitable for thin, irritable, tense, dyspeptic and dark patients. (If not helpful in a fair patient with the same history, try **Lobelia 30c**.)

Nux Vomica 30c. One dose every 15–30 minutes. Stop with improvement.

Brought on by extreme anger, indignation, humiliation or disappointment, particularly if the reaction is suppressed. Usually in a very sensitive person who takes offence easily. Pain as if brain were bruised; as if there was a heavy ball in the forehead; a bursting sensation; like a nail driven into the brain. Better after food, warmth and a night's sleep.

Staphysagria 30c. One dose every 15–30 minutes. Stop with improvement.

Periodic or Recurring

In conjunction with sudden respiratory infection, or after exposure to severe cold, with nasal discharge. Preceded by visual disturbances – double vision, blind spots, or flickering sight. Appears heavy and drowsy, with heaviness of eye-lids. Pain worse on first lying down but better later. Starts in back of neck and head, becomes a boring pain over front of head, usually worse over the right eye. Better for sleep. Worse for motion and light. Passes increased urine as pain ceases.

Gelsemium 30c or **200c**. Three doses, one in the morning, evening and following morning, a few days after the migraine, to prevent a recurrence.

Brought on by relaxing after mental strain, i.e. typical weekend headache. Preceded by one or two days of great lethargy and tiredness. Can sleep at any time. Usually wakened in early morning with nausea and vomiting, and a burning acid indigestion. Vomits white, sticky, stringy mucus. Frequently a watery, windy diarrhoea with a burning feeling in the anus. Violent headache, great heat and fullness, with a stupefying pain usually worse on the right side. Worse on being still. Better for continuous gentle movement. Cool air comforting but worse for cold draughts and after rest.

Iris Versicolor 30c. Three doses, one in the morning, evening and following morning, a few days after the migraine, to prevent a recurrence.

Congestion with aching; like many hammers hammering on the brain. On waking in the morning. After menstruation; sunrise to sunset. Sometimes one-sided. Eyes feel bruised. Nausea and vomiting. Preceded by visual disturbances or numbness and tingling in the lips, tongue and face. Chilly, depressed patients. Muscularly weak. Worse after grief, fright; with consolation; at seaside; heat. Better for open air, cold applications.

Natrum Muriaticum 30c. Three doses, one in the morning, evening and following morning, a few days after the migraine to prevent a recurrence.

Do not use this remedy during the headache. The acute phase is best treated by using **Apis**, **Bryonia** or **Ignatia**.

(*continued overleaf*)

HEADACHE AND MIGRAINE (continued)

Feeling as if the whole head were full to bursting, or that the eyes were being pushed outwards by the pressure. Pain starts in the back of the head and spreads forward; frequently worse on the right side. Sometimes a very changeable pattern of neuralgic pains in the face, teeth and upper jaw. Starts in the morning and lasts until the evening; clears with a night's sleep. Burning heat in palms and soles. Better lying in a dark room.

Sanguinaria 30c. Three doses, one in the morning, evening and following morning, a few days after the migraine, to prevent a recurrence.

Pulsating, throbbing and stabbing. Usually after an emotional problem, starting in the morning and easing away by evening. Starts at the back of head, moves over the top and settles over the left eye or left temple. Pain in the eyes, particularly the left eye, which feels too big for the socket. Stabbing pain back through the head with stiff neck and shoulders. Pain worse by noise, using the eyes and by any motion, especially jarring. Better by lying on the right side and propped up on pillows.

Spigelia 30c. Three doses, one in the morning, evening and following morning, a few days after the migraine, to prevent a recurrence.

HERPES – MOUTH OR GENITAL

You will have had this condition diagnosed by your doctor. For self-help it is worth trying **Rhus Toxicodendron 6c** three times a day at the first sign of itch or tingling. Continue with this for the duration of a recurrent attack.

HOARSENESS AND LOSS OF VOICE

Hoarseness and loss of voice are commonly associated with colds and flu's and with 'colds going down on to the chest'. Some people suffer more than others, and the problem may occur for no very obvious reason at all. In some occupations involving singing or speaking, hoarseness and loss of voice are an occupational hazard.

The homoeopathic remedies on the page opposite are useful as First Aid remedies. If the hoarseness persists for more than two to three weeks you should consult your own doctor. He will probably refer you to an Ear, Nose and Throat specialist for investigation to exclude other more serious disease. If nothing serious is found by the specialist, treatment by an experienced homoeopath is likely to be most beneficial.

HOARSENESS AND LOSS OF VOICE

Hoarseness with a sensation of rawness in the larynx. Worse with cough, swallowing or speaking. May have thick sputum.	**Argentum Metallicum 6c** or **Argentum Nitricum 6c.** One dose 2–4 times a day. Reduce with improvement.
Hoarseness after severe over-use, e.g. shouting, screaming, singing.	**Arnica 6c.** One dose 2–4 times a day. Reduce with improvement.
Variable hoarseness. Voice changes pitch, difficult to control. Hawking phlegm. Better resting. Worse singing and talking.	**Arum Triphyllum 6c.** One dose 2–4 times a day. Reduce with improvement.
Loss of voice after excessive use. Worse in the morning. Raw larynx. Better with cold drinks.	**Causticum 6c.** One dose 2–4 times a day. Reduce with improvement.
Hoarseness worse in the evening and early night. Larynx painful, preventing speech. Dry, tickling cough made worse moving into cold air.	**Phosphorus 6c.** One dose 2–4 times a day. Reduce with improvement.
Speaking and singing. Hoarseness at beginning; improves while using voice; hoarseness at end when tired.	**Rhus Toxicodendron 6c.** One dose 2–4 minutes before using voice.

INDIGESTION (DYSPEPSIA)

This is a state of discomfort in the lower chest and upper stomach, with some of the following complaints: a heavy sensation in the stomach after food; actual swelling of the stomach area; bloating – a sensation of swelling with or without flatulent 'wind' belched up or rumbling around, or trapped and uncomfortable; burping up watery or solid stomach contents; 'acidity' – sharp or burning pains in the upper abdomen.

These symptoms may arise in a number of different combinations, but acute attacks are short-lived and the cause can usually be avoided (e.g. by not eating particular foods or by eating in a more regular and relaxed way).

Chronic indigestion which has gone on for weeks, months or years should be investigated by your doctor, since treatment is less likely to be by means of simple measures, and there may be a more serious underlying condition.

One of the most common causes of long-lasting or recurring bouts of indigestion is psychological stress, and this is why homoeopathic remedies can be so helpful.

Constitutional treatment that addresses the psychological factors is most likely to be successful; however, the following remedies can be used in a First Aid way.

It goes without saying that diet, rest and relaxation must be improved. Where possible, stressful situations should be avoided. When this cannot be done, one must learn, by whatever means possible, to be less affected by stress. Most people try to avoid changing any established patterns of living and thinking. Remedies alone should not be expected to compensate for the bad habits of a lifetime. The remedies on the opposite page may be used at the onset of a bout of indigestion. Vary the frequency of the dose according to the patient's response, increasing the intervals between doses as the patient improves.

The remedies may also be used at a rate of two or three times a day for a few days to treat a more longstanding situation.

INDIGESTION (DYSPEPSIA)

Dyspepsia in a bleak, ill-looking, chilly and fussy person. Very poor appetite. May have diarrhoea.

Arsenicum Album 6c. One dose at intervals of 15–30 minutes for 2–3 doses.

Heavy weight in stomach immediately after food. Bitter taste. Nausea and pains through to back and shoulders. Headache.

Bryonia 6c. One dose at intervals of 15–30 minutes for 2–3 doses.

Belching wind and sour taste. Pain in pit of stomach. Generally worse after eating.

Carbo Vegetabilis 6c. One dose at intervals of 15–30 minutes for 2–3 doses.

Great flatulence and bowel rumbling. Unwell if meals missed or delayed. Likes sweet things.

Lycopodium 6c. One dose at intervals of 15–30 minutes for 2–3 doses.

Overeating. Irritability. Bloated, heavy feeling in stomach. Flatulence and heartburn. Sometimes nausea and vomiting. Too much alcohol.

Nux Vomica 6c. One dose at intervals of 15–30 minutes for 2–3 doses.

Changeable symptoms. Thirstless, coated tongue. Likes fats and rich foods – but they disagree and cause nausea. Full, bloated feeling two hours after food.

Pulsatilla 6c. One dose at intervals of 15–30 minutes for 2–3 doses.

Long history of dyspepsia. Sour belching. Constipation and bowel rumbling. Overeating and overdrinking.

Sulphur 6c. One dose at intervals of 15–30 minutes for 2–3 doses.

INFLAMMATION, BOILS AND ABSCESSES

Swelling, pain, tenderness and redness, commonly found on the outer parts of the body, is due to inflammation, and is caused by the defensive reactions of the body to infection by germs. These germs may enter through damaged skin; in a case of inflammation deep inside the body they may have been carried there by the blood stream. If the defensive reaction is successful the inflammation fades away; but if the reaction is weak, or the infection virulent, an abscess may form.

An abscess is a walled-off collection of pus which is a mixture of liquified dead blood cells, dead germs and nearby tissues. On the surface of the skin it forms the familiar rounded tense mass called a boil. Boils may also form when hair follicles become infected.

The natural healing process of an abscess is to form a head and then to discharge the pus. It is safe for a boil on the surface to do this, but it may not be safe for a deep abscess to do so, and antibiotics and surgical help will be needed. If your doctor diagnoses a deep abscess he will refer you to a surgeon; follow his or her advice. You can also use homoeopathic remedies to good effect at the same time.

A carbuncle is a raised, inflamed and infected area of the skin which has several heads or openings, each of which may discharge pus separately. This is a serious condition because it can spread and destroy areas of skin, and can cause a severe general illness. It is also serious because there may be an underlying condition needing diagnosis and treatment, such as diabetes mellitus.

It is essential that you consult your doctor for examination. It is almost certain that he will need to give you antibiotics. Again, you should take the appropriate homoeopathic remedies at the same time – there is no risk that they will work against each other.

The required homoeopathic remedies are divided into three groups, relating to the stages of: (i) Inflammation; (ii) Early formation; and (iii) Later formation and discharge of pus. There will tend to be some overlapping, but start at the stage which seems most appropriate, and change the remedy if the picture changes.

Use moist **Hypercal** dressings prepared by adding ten drops to a glass of cool, previously boiled water.

INFLAMMATION, BOILS AND ABSCESSES

Inflammation

Early, mild symptoms of inflammation. Slight redness and discomfort. No generalised illness.

Ferrum Phosphoricum 6c. One dose 3–4 times a day until better.

Skin easily infected. Sharp stabbing pain. Very tender and very sore. Prickling.

Early stage to stop development if possible. **Hepar Sulphuris 30c.** One dose every 4 hours until better.

Later stage to encourage boil to burst. **Hepar Sulphuris 6c.** One dose every 4 hours until better.

Early Formation

As above but also:

Shining and swollen. Pains sting and burn, worse with hot applications and better with cold ones.

Apis 6c. One dose 2–4 hours until better.

Bright red swelling. Hot throbbing pain, worse with cold applications and dressings. Feverish.

Belladonna 6c. One dose every 2–4 hours until better.

Blue or purple skin around area. Very tender. Worse with hot applications.

Lachesis 6c. One dose every 2–4 hours until better.

Later Formation and Discharge of Pus

Note all previous remedies.

Hot and cold with chills. Restless, anxious, confused. Rapid pulse and low temperature, or high temperature and slow pulse. **Consult your doctor**.

Pyrogen 6c. One dose every 2–4 hours until better.

Very rapid inflammation. Burning, stinging, throbbing pain. Very tender. Restless and anxious. **Consult your doctor**.

Tarentula Cubensis 30c. One dose every 2–4 hours until better.

INFLUENZA

Influenza is the name given to a very large number of viral infections which usually occur as epidemics, particularly in the cold winter months. It is often found that one or two specific homoeopathic remedies are useful for most of the victims of any particular outbreak.

Prevention is difficult, since the viruses are usually spread by coughs and sneezes in crowded places. However, the use of 'Colds and Flu' tablets (taken one in the morning and evening on the first and perhaps also on the fifteenth of each month) will act like an immunisation and build up the resistance of the patient.

The symptoms vary with each type of viral infection. Usually they divide into those that affect the nose, throat and chest and those that affect the stomach and the bowels. Both groups have general complaints of headaches, muscular aches and pains, and fevers. Some viruses can cause bleeding, such as nose bleeds, altered periods, or bruising of the skin (purpura).

The homoeopathic remedies on the page opposite are a few of the main remedies which will help with influenza. Choose the most similar symptom picture. If you cannot decide between two remedies you may give both of them alternately about one hour apart. Watch for changes in the symptoms of the patient and be prepared to change the remedy.

General Measures for Treatment

- For general measures to help the patient see also the sections for: 'Fevers', pages 96–7; 'Colds', pages 120–3; 'Diarrhoea', pages 132–3; 'Nausea and Vomiting', pages 164–5.
- Rest the patient, preferably in bed. The room should be warm and ventilated.
- Encourage the patient to drink as much fluid as possible. A light diet is usually preferred by patients – a little and often of what the patient fancies is usually best.

INFLUENZA

First Signs and Early Stages

At the very first signs of fever. Red, dry skin. Very thirsty for lots of cold drinks. Anxious, agitated. Sudden chill, shivering, from cold, dry winds.	**Aconite 30c.** One dose at intervals of one to two hours for 3–4 doses. If no better, proceed to another remedy.
Sudden very high fever. Very red face. Throbbing headache, may be delirious; Hates noise and bright light. May sweat, but usually has hot, *dry* skin.	**Belladonna 6c.** One dose at intervals of one to two hours. Stop with improvement.
Gradual onset of mild fever. Sweaty skin, pallor and flushing face. May have nosebleeds, earache, and painful tracheitis and cough (i.e. going down into chest).	**Ferrum Phosphoricum 6c.** One dose at intervals of one to two hours. Stop with improvement.
Sudden intense chill with shivering. Unable to get warm. Patient irritable. Nose dry and stuffed up.	**Nux Vomica 6c**. One dose at intervals of one to two hours. Stop with improvement.

Later Stages

Sweating. Lies very still as any movement intensifies headache and aches and pains. Very dry mouth and throat. Very great thirst for large drinks of cold water.	**Bryonia 6c.** One dose at intervals of two to three hours. Stop with improvement.
Back is sore, stiff and aching. Pain in the eyeballs; muscles and bones ache. Thirsty for cold drinks.	**Eupatorium Perfoliatum 6c.** One dose at intervals of two to three hours. Stop with improvement.
Red face and throbbing headache. Tired and drowsy; shivering. Aches in back, joint and limbs. Not thirsty. Wants to lie down and sleep.	**Gelsemium 6c.** One dose every two to three hours. Stop with improvement.
Aches and pains and stiffness, helped by restless movements. Sweating in bed – shivering if uncovered. Cold areas of body in spite of fever. Very thirsty for cold drinks. Cold sores in and around mouth (herpes).	**Rhus Toxicodendron 6c.** One dose every two to three hours. Stop with improvement.

IRRITABLE BOWEL SYNDROME (IBS)

The symptoms of irritable bowel syndrome are varied. They include alternating diarrhoea and constipation, abdominal distension with much rumbling, abdominal pains and the passing of much flatus.

Any change in bowel habit from the patient's normal pattern must be investigated by the doctor. The diagnosis of irritable bowel syndrome is made on the clinical history and by excluding other pathology – there is no distinct test for IBS.

IBS may be triggered by various factors, such as stress, food intolerances and a previous attack of gastroenteritis ('tummy bug').

The homoeopathic remedies listed opposite should be selected according to the symptoms.

IRRITABLE BOWEL SYNDROME (IBS)

Great flatulence with distension. Stool watery and windy. Worse after eating and drinking, and emotional stress, particularly anxiety in anticipation of an event.	**Argentum Nitricum 6c** or **30c.** One dose four times a day. Stop with improvement.
Diarrhoea from anxiety in anticipation, fright, bad news. Stool painless, cream or green. Generalised trembling and weakness.	**Gelsemium 6c** or **30c.** One dose four times a day. Stop with improvement.
Diarrhoea from fright, grief and disappointment. Trembling in hands. Griping pains in sides of abdomen. Spasmodic pain from anus up into rectum. Craves acid foods and drinks.	**Ignatia 30c** or **200c.** One dose four times a day. Stop with improvement.
Effects of anger and bad news. Anxiety, miserable, depressed. Usually constipated, but much belching of wind, abdominal distension, rumbling and colic. First stools lumpy and hard, then liquid, with passage of large volume of wind which improves discomfort. Better with local heat and hot drinks.	**Lycopodium 6c** or **30c.** One dose four times a day. Stop with improvement.
Effects of anger and resentment. Alternating constipation and diarrhoea, with abdominal colic and soreness, and uneasiness in rectum. Great relief after a bowel action. Stools either small and hard or loose, mixed with mucus and watery blood. Thick coated tongue. Nausea especially after food. Drowsy in daytime, especially after meals. Restless at night. Very irritable and sensitive to smells and noise.	**Nux Vomica 30c.** One dose four times a day. Stop with improvement.

MOUTH ULCERS (APHTHOUS ULCERS)

Most people suffer an occasional ulcer in the mouth, perhaps due to some minor injury from food or a toothbrush bristle. Some people have them in 'crops'. Occasionally, mouth ulcers may persist as a continuous problem for years, one or more developing as the previous one heals. They are very painful and can develop secondary infection. The cause is unknown – orthodox treatments tend to be many and varied, and generally unhelpful to most sufferers.

The homoeopathic remedies on the page opposite should help in the acute stages, and may reduce the severity and frequency of the ulcers. If you only have a few remedies available, **Rhus Toxicodendron** is likely to be one of them. If the condition is of long standing, or if the remedies do not help, consult a doctor for investigation and assessment. If there is no underlying medical problem, and your attempts at first aid have not been helpful, consult an experienced homoeopath.

MOUTH ULCERS (APHTHOUS ULCERS)

Small red vesicles becoming ulcers. Painful to touch; worse with acid or salty foods.	**Borax 6c.** One dose three times a day reducing with improvement.
Thick, sticky saliva. Tongue swollen. Ulcers especially on inside of lower lip. Cold sores on lower lip.	**Hydrastis 6c.** One dose three times a day, reducing with improvement.
Salivation increased, with metallic taste; but thirsty. Tongue soft and swollen. Bad breath. Shallow ulcers, burning pain. Neck glands may be tender and swollen.	**Mercurius Solubilis 6c.** One dose three times a day, reducing with improvement.
If Mercurius Solubilis is not effective. Ulcers with irregular edges tending to bleed easily. Stinging, pricking pain.	**Nitric Acid 6c.** One dose three times a day, reducing with improvement.
Tongue red and cracked, or white with a red tip. Gums sore, blisters turning to ulcers. Ulcerated corners of mouth, cold sores on lips.	**Rhus Toxicodendron 6c.** One dose three times a day, reducing with improvement.

Oral Treatment

Tincture of **Hydrastis** in half a glass of cool, previously boiled water can be used as a mouth wash, as can **Hypercal** or **Calendula** tinctures. Sucking the remedy tablets will also act as local treatment.

NAUSEA AND VOMITING

Everyone is familiar with these symptoms. Nausea may be caused by irritation of the stomach, by infection or overeating and drinking. It may be part of the picture of a particular disease like influenza (pages 158–9), or a condition like pregnancy (pages 54–61). It may be caused by a disturbance of the organ of balance in the ear, as in travel sickness (pages 200–1), or in a specific condition like Menière's disease.

Vomiting occurs when the stomach contents are more or less violently forced up and out of the mouth. Occasionally vomiting occurs suddenly and for no obvious reason, and must then be investigated.

The homoeopathic remedies opposite are a few of a very long list, and should help in most cases.

Care must be taken to prevent dehydration due to vomiting in children, and especially in babies. This is particularly important in very hot weather. Feeding small quantities of water (a little and often), or getting the baby to sip from a teaspoon, should prevent this.

If there is any doubt your doctor should be consulted urgently, or the infant taken to the local hospital.

NAUSEA AND VOMITING

No appetite, belching. Tongue coated thick and white. Irritable and complaining.

Antimonium Crudum 6c. One dose at intervals of 1–2 hours. Reduce with improvement.

Burning pain and acid vomiting. Coldness, chills and weakness. Great anxiety. Frequently diarrhoea also.

Arsenicum Album 6c. One dose at intervals of 1–2 hours. Reduce with improvement.

Intense nausea and sweating. No relief from vomiting. Tongue remains clean, profuse saliva. May have diarrhoea also.

Ipecacuanha 6c. One dose at intervals of 1–2 hours. Reduce with improvement.

Bloated, heavy feeling in stomach. Belching, heartburn. 'Dietary indiscretion' and overeating. Worse in morning and after food. Hypersensitive, irritable, fastidious. 'Morning after the night before'. Hangover.

Nux Vomica 6c. One dose at intervals of 1–2 hours. Reduce with improvement.

NETTLE RASH (HIVES, URTICARIA)

This is a skin condition where there is a rapid, but usually short lived, appearance of wheals on the skin surface, together with a burning, stinging or tingling sensation. The wheals are variable in size and shape, and consist of a central white area surrounded by reddened skin. The patient may suffer from general malaise, anxiety or fear, and a raised temperature.

In other words it looks and feels much like the sting of the common stinging nettle.

It has a variety of causes, being an allergic or sensitivity reaction to:

- Chemicals (detergents, garden sprays, scents)
- Drugs (antibiotics, aspirin)
- Insect bites or stings (bees, wasps)
- Plant and fruit juices (primulas, strawberries)
- Foods (eggs, shellfish, nuts)

Occasionally acute anxiety or fear may bring about nettle rash, in a person who is predisposed to it.

However, nettle rash is the outward show of a generalised reaction, because the cause is an imbalance of one of the defence mechanisms of the body.

General Treatment

The cause or causes of any episode must be discovered, e.g. bee stings, a particular food or drink. This particular cause must then be carefully avoided in future. Of course this may not be easy, especially during travels away from home. Find out which remedy or remedies listed opposite help, and then always carry them with you.

NETTLE RASH (HIVES, URTICARIA)

Raised blotchy rash with white centres. Violent itching with burning and numbness, worse with cold. In the later stage, there may be swelling of lips and eyelids.	**Urtica Urens 6c** or **30c.** One dose every 10–20 minutes. Reduce with improvement.
(This is generally the most useful remedy.)	
Burning, itching redness and swelling. Sensation of pins and needles or ants crawling under the skin. Angioedema. Very acute cases with much general swelling as well as the rash. Restlessness, anxiety, even fear.	**Agaricus 6c**. One dose every 10–20 minutes. Stop with improvement.
Swollen rash, especially from insect stings. Can extend over whole body. Itching worse at night. Pain is stinging and burning. Very sensitive. Worse from local warmth and pressure. Swellings of face, lips and eyelids.	**Apis 6c** or **30c.** One dose every 10–20 minutes. Reduce with improvement.
Blotchy raised rash with fever. Violent itching, burning pain. Rash may turn to blisters.	**Copaiva 6c.** One dose every 10–20 minutes. Reduce with improvement.
Prickling, tickling rash – turning to burning after scratching. Worse in evening. Better for local warmth. Rash may turn to blisters.	**Rhus Toxicodendron 6c.** One dose every 10–20 minutes. Reduce with improvement.

(*Note:* See 'Insect Bites and Stings', pages 22–3.)

OPERATIONS

The effects of surgical operations on most patients are similar, and fairly standard treatments can be offered.

Care Before Operation

Anxiety before admission to hospital, and before operation, can be eased by several remedies. (See also 'Anxiety', pages 108–9.) The three most likely to be helpful are indicated on the opposite page. The remedy chosen can be taken before going to bed for the few nights before going to hospital.

Prevention of Bleeding. Some people bleed readily. Dental and nose and throat operations tend to cause quick bleeding.

Arnica taken before and after the operation tends to reduce bleeding and bruising. For people with a bleeding tendency, or for operations in a region known to bleed freely, **Phosphorus** is the remedy of choice.

Pain, Bruising and Swelling. These are usual after operations. If **Arnica** and **Hypericum** are taken together, before and after the operation, all the unpleasant side effects will be greatly reduced, and far fewer pain-relieving drugs will be required.

Shock. The shock that surgery may produce will be greatly reduced by having taken **Arnica** beforehand.

There will be no reaction between homoeopathic remedies and the drugs which the hospital medical staff may have to prescribe. When in hospital it is quite possible that the staff will insist that you should not take any other medicines than the ones you are given. This will include homoeopathic remedies. If this is so, there is very little you can do. Please remember that the staff have a legal responsibility for patients in their care, and they must be allowed to conduct treatment as they judge best.

Allergies. Remember to tell the doctors and nurses about known allergies and any adverse reactions you may have had to previous anaesthetics and pain-relieving drugs.

OPERATIONS

Care Before Operation

Anxiety

Anxiety, excited, agitated. Hurried speech and behaviour. Restless – one unfinished activity after another.

Argentum Nitricum 30c. One dose for insomnia, and before admission and operation.

Anxious. Poor memory. Confused. Weak and trembling. Tendency to diarrhoea.

Gelsemium 30c. One dose for insomnia, and before admission and operation.

Emotional; oversensitive. Self-centred; changeable moods. Easily distracted from problems. Hysterical behaviour and gestures. Sighing.

Ignatia 30c. One dose a day for a few days before admission.

Prevention of Bleeding

Phosphorus 6c. One dose morning and evening the day before; and one dose the morning of the operation.

Pain, Bruising and Swelling. Shock

Arnica 6c or **30c** and **Hypericum 6c.** One dose of each taken together three times a day the day before operation and continued through the recovery period.

(*continued overleaf*)

OPERATIONS (continued)

Care After Operation

Drowsiness and confusion after the operation are usual in most people for a day or so, but they are more pronounced in some cases. Occasionally this state can last for several days. If this happens (or happened after a previous operation) **Opium 30c** may be of help, taken on the first day after the operation.

Nausea and vomiting (see pages 164–5).

Bleeding which arises after the operation must obviously be attended to by the surgical and nursing staff, but also take **Phosphorus 6c** as indicated.

Pain, bruising and swelling will continue to be controlled by taking **Arnica 6c** and **Hypericum 6c**.

Flatulence and wind which will not pass either up or down causes painful swelling of the stomach and bowels. If this develops, use **Raphanus 6c**.

Physical weakness, faintness and general lack of 'get up and go' will be helped by **China 6c**, three or four times a day, for the first few days after the operation.

'Nervous exhaustion' which develops after operation with some people can be helped by **Kali Phosphoricum 30c**, three or four times a day for a few days, and then twice a day for about a week as recovery occurs.

OPERATIONS (continued)

Care After Operation

Pain, bruising and swelling.	**Arnica 6c** and **Hypericum 6c.** One dose of each together three to four times a day for 3–4 days.
Physical weakness. Faintness. Lack of 'get up and go'. Loss of fluids (sweating, bleeding, vomiting).	**China 6c.** One dose 4 times a day for about one week.
Hypersensitive, irritable, moody. Insomnia. Nervous exhaustion. Weakness. Easily tired. Poor concentration. Unable to get back to work.	**Kali Phosphoricum 30c.** One dose morning and evening for 7–10 days.
Drowsiness, confusion. Especially after a long anaesthetic. Difficulty in waking up.	**Opium 30c.** One dose two or three times on the first day after operation.
Bleeding and oozing of blood.	**Phosphorus 6c.** One dose two or three times on the first day after operation.
Flatulence, wind. Swollen painful abdomen. Unable to pass wind.	**Raphanus 6c.** One dose at intervals of 1–2 hours until relief.

PAIN

Pains of many kinds are discussed throughout this book under the sections on the particular conditions in which they may arise. This present section is intended to serve as a general summary of different kinds of pain and the homoeopathic remedies which may bring relief. Homoeopathic remedies are very effective in reducing or removing pain in most problems, but the remedy must be accurately chosen.

Usually patients have great difficulty in describing the quality of the pain which is affecting them, and even more in working out what makes it better or worse.

Things to bear in mind are:

- The site – the organ or limb; left or right side.
- The quality – burning, stabbing, cramping, smarting, stinging, shooting.
- The direction – within, outward, upward, downward, side to side, diagonally, wandering, radiating.
- Other related symptoms – such as sweating, vomiting, restlessness, anxiety.
- Modalities – better or worse for time of day or night; hot or cold weather; wet or dry weather; the effect of thunder and lightning; local heat or cold; touch and pressure; stillness or movement.

The following types of pain are by no means exhaustive but occur commonly. Apply the descriptions to your problem and if necessary check the modalities by using local heat, pressure or movement and so on, in order to get increasing accuracy.

PAIN

Aching, Bruised and Sore

Aches, bruised soreness of muscles after trauma and overexercise. Bruising and stiffness. Sensation that bed is too hard. Worse by touch, movement and damp cold.	**Arnica 6c** or **30c.** One dose 2–4 times a day until improvement.
Muscular stiffness and aching pain. Prostration and mental confusion. Drowsy. Agitated and fidgeting. Desires cold water. Unpleasant smell to sweat, urine, stools etc. and aching.	**Baptisia 6c.** One dose every 2–4 hours until improvement.
Body stiffness severe and pain in the bones. Agitation but movement aggravates. Pain in eyeballs with pressure. Thirst for cold water.	**Eupatorium Perfoliatum 6c.** One dose at intervals of 1–2 hours until improvement.
Septic conditions Sore bruised sensation – bed too hard. Painful bones. All secretions smell putrid. Pulse rapid with low fever, or fever high and pulse low. Anxiety and agitation. Relief by changing position.	**Pyrogen 6c.** One dose every 2–4 hours until improvement in acute cases. In long continued cases give **Pyrogen 6c** one dose in morning and **Silica 6c** one dose in evening.
Rheumatism of joints, after exercise Stiff joints; aching soreness. Better by slow movement and changes in position, local heat and hot dry weather. Worse by cold damp weather and contact with moisture; by rest; by the beginning of movement and tiredness.	**Rhus Toxicodendron 6c** or **30c.** One at start of pain and repeat with its return, or one morning and evening. Reduce with improvement.

Burning

Burning with red swelling, with a pricking sensation. Stinging. Worse by heat, better by cold. In fever, dry skin; no thirst.	**Apis 6c.** One dose every 15–30 minutes. Reduce with improvement.

(*continued overleaf*)

PAIN (continued)

Intense burning pain helped by warmth. Worse at night between midnight and 3 a.m. Thirst for small frequent drinks. Anxiety, fear, agitation. Weakness, prostration, pallor.

Arsenicum Album 6c. One dose every 2–4 hours depending on the severity of symptoms. Reduce with improvement.

Severe burning in the bladder and urethra, before, during and after passing urine. Only a few drops of urine – dark and bloody. Large, tender, burning, itching blisters helped by cold applications. Better for warmth and hot applications. Second degree burns.

Cantharis 6c. One dose 2–4 times a day depending on the severity. Reduce with improvement.

Burning with tenderness in the mucous membranes, which are very dry and raw, as if scalded. Worse every seven days, and in daytime.

Sanguinaria 6c. One dose 2–3 times a day. Reduce with improvement.

Burning, itching of the skin, worse from washing and heat of bed. Better by cold. Usually caused by skin problems – acne, eczema, psoriasis etc.

Sulphur 6c. One dose morning and evening. (see 'Eczema', pages 134–5). Reduce with improvement.

Cramping, Spasmodic, Colicky

Unbearable pain with engorgement. Worse from 9 p.m. to midnight, by reprimand in children, or anger. Better for warmth (except toothache). Teething, earache and colic in infants. Better by being carried or driven.

Chamomilla 6c. One dose every 10 minutes. Reduce with improvement. Stop when pain ceases.

Spasmodic cramps in the digestive and female systems and neuralgic pains in the face and sciatic region. Makes patient scream out. Worse with cold. Better for firm pressure and bending double.

Colocynthis 6c or **30c**. One dose every 10–15 minutes. Reduce with improvement.

Spasmodic pain starting and ending suddenly. Cramps in calves and feet, especially in the elderly. Worse at night and for touch and pressure.	**Cuprum Metallicum 6c.** For night cramps, one dose before retiring. For other cramps, one dose at 10-minute intervals.
Paroxysms of colicky abdominal pains; twisting or crushing nature. Better bending backwards.	**Dioscorea 6c.** One dose every 10–15 minutes. Reduce with improvement.
Muscular spasms of neck, limbs, back and throat, in tense and hypersensitive people. Spasms of the face. Pains flitting, erratic and very localised. Frequently caused by reaction to unhappy events such as mourning, anxiety, accidents, disappointed love, emotional shock.	**Ignatia 6c.** One dose morning and evening. Reduce with improvement *or* **Ignatia 30c.** One dose night, morning and next night. Repeat every few days.
Severe cramp-like or neuralgic pain. Erratic. Sudden beginning and end. Usually on right side. Better for heat and bending forward in abdominal pain.	**Magnesium Phosphoricum 6c.** One dose every 2–4 hours. Reduce with improvement.

Pricking, Splinter-like

Piles – rectal skin dry and congested; raw and sore. Rectum feels as if full of needles. Lumbar backache – sacroiliac joints. Worse during sleep and standing; with heat. Better with cold and moderate exercise.	**Aesculus Hippocastanum 6c.** One dose 2–3 times a day. Reduce with improvement.
Itching skin, pricked by needles. Feeling as though skin frozen. Tremor and shivering.	**Agaricus 30c.** One dose twice a day. Reduce with improvement.
Tonsillitis, pharyngitis, laryngitis. Prickly sensation in the throat, vagina, urethra, stomach etc. Worse for heat, anxiety, sweet things. Better for fresh air and pressure on the painful area.	**Argentum Nitricum 6c.** One dose 2–3 times a day. Reduce with improvement.

(continued overleaf)

PAIN (continued)

Hypersensitive to pain, touch and cold air; irritable and easily angered. Needle or fishbone sensation. Boils and spots sensitive to cold and touch. Long term enlargement of glands. Worse by cold, cold draughts, and touch. Better for warmth.

Hepar Sulphuris
6c. One dose 3–4 times a day.
30c. One dose a day.
Reduce with improvement.

Ulcers and fissures at border of mouth and anus; yellow skin. Plantar warts with yellow tinge. Bleeding soft warts. Pricking pain as from a needle or pin.

Nitric Acid 6c. One dose twice a day. Reduce with improvement.

Skin unhealthy and easily infected. Yellow nails, deformed and brittle; white spots. Pain like needles or nails driven in. Feet cold and sweaty, and smell offensive.

Silica 6c. One dose morning and evening.

Shooting

Throbbing pain with additional shooting pains; starting and ending suddenly. Redness and congestion, with hot sweats.

Belladonna 6c or **30c.*** One dose every 2–4 hours. More frequently in acute states.

Rounded rash on the skin. Spasmodic shooting, burning pains; localised. Especially left-sided renal colic, worse for deep pressure. Urinary symptoms present also.

Berberis 6c or **30c.*** One dose every 10–20 minutes. Reduce with improvement.

Severe, erratic and shooting pains. Cramp-like pains with muscular stiffness and twitching. Uterine pain during periods – worse with increased flow.

Cimicifuga 6c or **30c.*** One dose 2–4 times a day. Reduce with improvement.

*In the acute situation the remedy should be given immediately the pain starts and be repeated as frequently as needed. Increase the time interval with improvement.

Shooting pains down length of the affected nerve. Worse for touch and movement. All injuries to nerves, skin, fingertips, toes and nails. Painful scars. Tooth extractions.

Hypericum 30c or **200c.***

Short-term treatment
One dose every 4–6 hours. Reduce with improvement.

Long-term treatment
One dose morning and evening.

Shooting pains in the nerves especially of the head, face and left chest wall. Left-sided trigeminal neuralgia. Worse for cold and wet; movement and touch. Headache worse for heat.

Spigelia 6c or **30c.*** One dose morning and evening. Reduce with improvement.

Stabbing, Stitching, Lancinating

Sudden severe neuralgia in any part, especially the face. Caused by sudden exposure to dry, frosty, cold wind. Pains sudden, unbearable, frightening; may alternate with numbness or pins and needles.

Aconite 30c. One dose every 2–4 hours. Reduce with improvement.

Sudden severe piercing pains. Worse by the least movement or touch; warm room. Better for local heat, continuous pressure and rest; by lying on painful side; by sweating.

Bryonia 30c. One dose every 2–4 hours. Reduce with improvement.

Sudden severe piercing pains. Distressing; a feeling of internal ulcers. Worse by touch and slightest movement; by change in weather and temperature; by wet cold weather. Blisters contain a bloody liquid.

Ranunculus Bulbosus 30c. One dose every 2–4 hours. Reduce with improvement.

Neuralgic stabbing pains of head and chest wall, especially trigeminal neuralgia and left-sided migraine. Skin tender and swollen over painful area.

Spigelia 6c or **30c.** One dose every 2–4 hours. Reduce with improvement.

(*continued overleaf*)

PAIN (continued)

Stinging, Smarting

Swelling and itching. Burning, stinging, smarting. Worse for heat and touch. Better for cold.

Apis 6c. One dose every 10–15 minutes. Reduce with improvement.

Severe, piercing, stinging pain. Worse for the least movement or touch and by hot rooms and hot weather. Better for continuous pressure, local heat and by rest, or lying on affected side. Intense thirst in fever.

Bryonia 6c or **30c.** Up to three times a day. Reduce with improvement.

Wounds due to cut of knife (surgical incisions; see 'Operations', pages 168–71). Prostatic symptom of a drop of urine constantly in the urethra.

Staphysagria 6c or **30c.** One dose morning and evening. Reduce with improvement.

Honeymoon cystitis.

Staphysagria 30c. One dose every 4–6 hours. Alternate with **Cantharis 6c.** Reduce with improvement.

Itching, burning, stinging. Better for local heat. Worse by cold bathing or washing. Urticaria.

Urtica Urens 6c. One dose every 2–4 hours. Reduce with improvement.

Throbbing, Pulsating

Face red and congested. Temperature about 39°C or 40°C. Hot sweats, especially on face. Throbbing headache. Scarlet fever-like rash. Delirious. Convulsions or nearly comatose.

Belladonna 6c or **30c.** One dose at intervals of 1–2 hours. Reduce with improvement.

Throbbing headache. Hypersensitive skin and scalp. Buzzing in ears and partial deafness.

China 6c or **30c.** One dose morning and evening. Reduce with improvement.

Congestion of face. Sunstroke. Throbbing expanding headaches, in time with heart beat. Fullness of neck. Worse by heat; being jolted, constricting clothes, ties etc. Better in open air; holding head firmly.

Glonoinum 6c or **30c.** One dose immediately, then 2–3 times a day until improvement.

Hot flushes, throbbing migraines, usually left sided. Worse by heat; before the period. Better by discharges – menstrual periods, vomiting. Bored, jealous, vindictive and suspicious. Skin hypersensitive.

Lachesis 6c or **30c.** One dose every 2–4 hours. Reduce with improvement.

PERSPIRATION – EXCESSIVE

Excessive generalised perspiration may be due to hot weather, hot airless surroundings indoors, or to exertion. The treatment is then obvious.

But 'hot' perspiration may also be due to fever (e.g. influenza) or more rare illnesses such as excess thyroid secretion (thyrotoxicosis) or tuberculosis or occasionally to a malignancy. The 'hot flushes' of the menopause can give rise to profuse 'hot' perspiration, but acute anxiety states (see the sections on 'Anxiety' and 'Fear') usually, but not always, give rise to 'cold' perspiration, as does hypoglycaemia (low blood sugar).

The sweating may also occur in local areas, e.g. upper lip, forehead, head and scalp, body, armpits, groin, palms and soles, and may be sweet, salty or offensive in spite of otherwise adequate hygiene.

External Treatment

General

- Bath or shower morning and evening.
- Daily change of cotton underwear and more frequent change of shirts or blouses. Avoid man-made fibres if possible.

Feet

- Wash and dry feet at least once a day.
- Avoid heavy socks.
- Wear sandals if possible, rather than heavy shoes.

PERSPIRATION – EXCESSIVE

Cold, clammy, flabby, overweight. Sweating worse with exertion and humidity. Better for dry climate. Head sweats worse at night.	**Calcarea Carbonica 6c** or **30c.** One dose 2–3 times a day until improvement.
Profuse sour smelling sweat, especially on head. Itching. Worse for warmth. Better for cold and walking.	**Fluoric Acid 6c** or **30c.** One dose 2–3 times a day until improvement.
Greasy, offensive perspiration, especially feet and arm pits. Great itching of dry skin. Chronic eczema. Worse for warmth. Better for being cool.	**Lycopodium 6c** or **30c.** One dose 2–3 times a day until improvement.
Profuse sticky perspiration which does not relieve symptoms. Worse for warmth, night, damp weather.	**Mercurius Solubilis 6c** or **30c.** One dose 2–3 times a day until improvement.
Thin, chilly, anxious. Cold sweaty feet – very unpleasant smell. Soreness of feet.	**Silica 6c** or **30c.** One dose 2–3 times a day until improvement.
Red, dry, scaly skin. Offensive sweat. Itching. Sweaty hands and armpits, groin. Worse for warmth and washing. Better for dry conditions.	**Sulphur 6c** or **30c.** One dose 2–3 times a day until improvement.

PILES (HAEMORRHOIDS)

Piles are veins just inside the anus which begin to bulge and enlarge, and eventually to extrude or 'prolapse'. Initially the extruded or prolapsed piles return on their own, but they may eventually need to be pushed back after each motion has passed.

In Western countries the main cause of piles in both men and women is likely to be the low fibre content of the diet, causing some degree of constipation, although a bout of severe diarrhoea may also produce piles. A particular cause in women is the pressure of the baby during pregnancy and the force of straining in confinement. There can also be a family tendency to have piles.

The treatment of piles must be based on a diet containing adequate fibre, and this is best obtained from natural and unrefined foods. Sometimes an increase in liquids is needed as well.

Use the appropriate homoeopathic remedy. If the piles are prolapsed and painful the use of liquid paraffin (medicinal paraffin) for a few days can be helpful in softening the individual motions. The dose varies with the patient, but it is useful to start with one teaspoonful with the main meals and vary according to the results. *Do not continue the use of medicinal paraffin for more than one or two weeks.*

Caution

If you have used suitably chosen remedies and improved your diet and bowel habit over a month or two, and there has still been no improvement with the piles, or if they seem to be worse, consult a doctor.

But if the piles suddenly appear for no very obvious reason, or if they gradually enlarge, protrude and bleed, or if you develop a change of bowel habit, or at any time pass blood or mucus with the motions, **then you must consult your doctor immediately**. He will assess the situation, and decide if investigations are needed to exclude any serious disease, and what other methods of treatment ought to be considered.

PILES (HAEMORRHOIDS)

Piles: purple and bruised-looking. Splinter-like feeling in rectum. Anus dry, itching and burning. Low back pain.	**Aesculus Hippocastanum 6c.** One dose morning and evening. Reduce with improvement.
Piles: protruding like grapes. Bleeding. Scraped, burning sensation. Better for bathing with cold water.	**Aloe 6c.** One dose morning and evening. Reduce with improvement.
Piles: large, burning and stinging. Worse at night. Irritability. Constipated, small stools and a 'never finished' feeling.	**Nux Vomica 6c.** One dose morning and evening. Reduce with improvement.
Constipation, or a loose early-morning motion. Anal itching. Fullness, little bleeding. Headache and constipation.	**Sulphur 6c.** One dose morning and evening. Reduce with improvement.

It can be very difficult to decide which remedy is most likely to be effective, and indeed several others are possible. In this case take Nux Vomica 6c at night on retiring and Sulphur 6c first thing in the morning for one or two weeks.

External Treatment

Apply one or other of the following ointments night and morning, or after each motion: **Hamamelis, Aesculus Hippocastanum** or **Paeonia** (see page 213 under 'Ointments and Creams'). Although it is sometimes very difficult to do, washing after each bowel action helps to control itching and soreness. A spray bidet can be especially helpful.

PSORIASIS

This is the name given to a long-term skin condition which may arise in childhood, although usually later, with patches of thickening skin, crusting and scaling, and sometimes cracking and bleeding fissures.

It can occur on any area of the skin, but is typically found on the knees, elbows and in the scalp. Great thickness of the skin is typical of the elbows and knees, sometimes with cracking and bleeding. The scalp is more usually the site of great scaling, like severe dandruff.

Psoriasis tends to run in families, and sometimes seems to be brought about by excessive anxiety and stress. If this is thought to play a part, it is important to consult a homoeopath, because a thorough assessment of the family background and the psychological and physical make-up of the patient will be essential. Even so, treatment is likely to take several months.

ROSACEA (ACNE ROSACEA)

This is an abnormal reaction of the skin of the face, which eventually gives rise to a reddening and thickening of the skin. It covers the cheeks and sometimes the forehead. There is initially a variable flushing which gradually becomes more constant, with later prominent blood vessels, and later still, red, thickened skin and small spots.

There is frequently a sensation of burning and stinging, which is intensified by hot drinks and alcohol. It is most frequent in women at the menopause, but can occur in alcoholics of either sex. Rosacea is particularly disturbing since it so often comes with all the other problems of the menopausal age.

If the patient is very disturbed psychologically, and the suggested remedies provide insufficient relief, consult an experienced homoeopath, who will ensure that the constitutional homoeopathic treatment is given.

PSORIASIS

Fine, dry, scaling patches of skin. Burning, itching improved by local warmth.

Arsenicum Album 6c. One dose morning and evening. Reduce with improvement.

Leathery skin with rough, thickened and cracking patches. Nails thickened, splitting and pitted. Worse in winter.

Petroleum 6c. One dose morning and evening. Reduce with improvement.

Bloodstained fissures and cracks in very thickened skin patches. Itching not relieved by scratching.

Sepia 6c. One dose morning and evening. Reduce with improvement.

ROSACEA (ACNE ROSACEA)

Red, flushed skin. Granular appearance. Enlarged veins. Very symmetrical areas on cheeks and central forehead.

Arnica 6c. One dose morning and evening. Reduce with improvement.

Red, burning, stinging areas on the cheeks made worse by local heat. Hot flushes with red cheeks.

Sanguinaria 6c. One dose morning and evening. Reduce with improvement.

The treatment may have to be continued for several weeks.

External Treatment

This should be gentle. On no account should ointments or creams containing cortisone-type drugs be used. Applications of **Hamamelis** cream may be used, depending upon the individual response.

SHINGLES (HERPES ZOSTER)

Shingles is a very painful skin rash which follows the route of a nerve in the skin, and is caused by the chickenpox virus. The skin becomes inflamed, painful and tender so that movement, and even the touch of clothes, is intolerable. The variably-sized areas of inflammation develop several types of blisters which then burst and form dry scabs. Any area of the body surface can be affected. The head and face can be particularly troublesome.

If the eye is affected you must consult your own doctor. He or she will probably refer you to an eye specialist.

The aching or neuralgic shooting pains usually start before the skin rash appears, which can give rise to difficulties in diagnosis. If there is any doubt your family doctor should be consulted.

During all this time the patient is usually very unwell, with general aches, pains, malaise and some fever, and may have to go to bed.

General Treatment

- Stay off work.
- Bed rest is usually needed in the early stages, although some people may feel better for being up and about.
- The skin may have to be protected from contact with clothes. Some patients find **Calendula** ointment spread on sterile dressings very soothing, although if this is kept in position too long the skin may become soggy.
- The oozing from the blisters can be dressed by placing Melolin dressings over each area. Melolin is less likely to stick to the skin and absorbs the discharge.
- Oozing in the beard, scalp and hairy skin is best not dressed, but left alone for as long as possible. Sponging with a solution of **Calendula** or **Hypercal** tincture may help, 5ml (twenty drops) to 200ml (half a pint) of cool, previously boiled water.
- Try to reduce the pain by covering or applying hot or cold compresses to the shingles. Sometimes keeping very still (or moving about) will help the pain. If you find out what can improve (or worsen) the pain, this will help you to choose a remedy.

SHINGLES (HERPES ZOSTER)

Early treatment is important if severe neuralgic pains are to be prevented or reduced. The appearance of the rash and the things which aggravate or relieve the pain are of importance in choosing the remedy. If you find that your pain is not helped by your choice of remedy, alternate the two most likely remedies.

Large blisters with surrounding swelling. Burns, stings, prickles. Relieved by cool compresses.	**Apis 6c.** One dose four times a day while the blisters last.
Severe itching, burning pain, may be worse after midnight. Pain relieved by hot compresses. Restless, anxious, sleepless.	**Arsenicum Album 6c.** One dose four times a day while the blisters last.
Bluish blisters with bloodstained fluid. Itching. Touch and movement causes shocks and stabs of pain. Pain reduced by stillness and rest.	**Ranunculus Bulbosus 6c.** One dose four times a day while the blisters last.
Very small blisters with clear fluid. Pain and itching helped by restless movement. Hot compresses may relieve the pain.	**Rhus Toxicodendron 6c.** One dose four times a day while the blisters last.

If your first-aid treatment has not proved effective within a week, consult an experienced homoeopath without further delay.

SHINGLES, PAIN AFTER (POST-HERPETIC NEURALGIA)

One of the problems of shingles is the development of various pains in the area of the original blisters at the onset of the illness and after the blisters have cleared. These vary greatly from severe aching to sharp shooting and to intense burning.

Quite often the pains are bizarre and very variable (paraesthesia).

Most cases of post-herpetic neuralgia last only a few weeks but some persist for months and occasionally for many years. Orthodox treatment, especially in the elderly, is on the whole not very helpful for longstanding post-herpetic neuralgia, but treatment of the shingles by homoeopathic remedies generally reduces its severity and duration.

Use the remedy on the opposite page which you think is the most appropriate. If the problem persists consult an experienced homoeopath.

SHINGLES, PAIN AFTER (POST-HERPETIC NEURALGIA)

Raw burning sensation, worse at 3 a.m. and in dry cold. Better in rainy humid weather.	**Causticum 6c** or **30c.** One dose 3–4 times a day. Reduce with improvement.
Shooting pains along the length of a nerve; worse by movement or by contact with clothes.	**Hypericum 30c.** One dose 3–4 times a day and at onset of pain. Reduce with improvement.
Severe pain like electric shocks, from the centre outwards. Followed by swelling and tenderness. Worse with movement. Useful for neuralgia of the face and round the right eye.	**Kalmia Latifolia 30c.** One dose 3–4 times a day and at onset of pain. Reduce with improvement.
Spasms of pain, sudden, cramplike and unbearable, causing the patient to scream. Start and finish suddenly. Better with local heat.	**Magnesium Phosphoricum 30c.** One dose 3–4 times a day and at onset of pain. Reduce with improvement.
Severe prickly burning pains. Skin tender and swollen over painful area.	**Spigelia 30c.** One dose 3–4 times a day and at onset of pain. Reduce with improvement.

SINUSITIS AND CATARRH

The nasal sinuses are bony cavities found:

- on either side of the nose in the cheeks (maxillary sinuses)
- just above the root of the nose and over the inner roof of the eyes (frontal sinuses; these are smaller)
- at the back of the upper part of the nose (ethmoid sinuses)

They are all lined with a moist mucous membrane which is the same as the membranes of the trachea and the bronchi into the lungs.

Acute Sinusitis

When a patient gets an upper respiratory tract infection, all the parts of the system may be affected – nose, sinuses, throat, larynx, trachea and bronchi, and the lungs, and so initial treatment is of a typical cold or influenza – see 'Common Cold – Early Stages' (pages 120–1) and 'Influenza' (pages 158–9).

Longstanding Sinusitis

This is often due to the presence of polyps or bony malformations, which give rise to inadequate drainage of discharge. There is often great damage to the mucous membranes of the sinus or sinuses, caused by the combination of lack of drainage, infections, and large quantities of pus-like discharge. To prescribe homoeopathic remedies, consider any type of pain and its distribution, and the type of catarrh, together with those physical conditions which either worsen or improve them.

The type of discharge may be a very important guide, e.g.

- yellow
- green
- yellow/green
- bloody
- watery
- thick and stringy.

SINUSITIS AND CATARRH

Sticky mucus down back of throat, difficult to clear. Pain over root or bridge of nose, like heavy spectacles. There may be redness of the eye. Pain either frontal and worse with pressure, or around the eyes and shooting to temporal areas. Worse with extremes of temperature and at night.	**Cinnabaris 6c** or **30c.** One dose morning and evening. Stop with improvement.
Yellow discharge. Splinter-like pains in bones of face; very sensitive to touch and cold draught. Better in damp warmth.	**Hepar Sulphuris 6c.** One dose morning, noon and evening (increases discharge). Stop with improvement.
Worse from dry cold draughts and touch.	**Hepar Sulphuris 30c.** One dose twice daily. The higher potency will reduce the discharge.
Discharge of thick, sticky, stringy yellow or greenish-yellow mucus; can be bloodstained. Forms crusts in nose or a post-nasal drip causing frequent throat clearing. Better from local heat. Worse in the morning and in hot weather.	**Kali Bichromicum 6c** or **30c.** One dose morning and evening. Stop with improvement.
Intense pain over eyes and root of nose. Profuse, hot, watery nasal discharge – goes on either to dry nose or to thicker greenish discharge.	**Kali Iodatum 6c.** One dose 4 times a day. Stop with improvement.
Intense pain when the pus-like discharge stops due to the blockage of the sinuses. Pain better when flow starts again. Mottled purple swelling over affected sinus. Worse after sleep and from pressure. Better for local warmth.	**Lachesis 30c.** One dose 4 times a day. Stop with improvement.

(*continued overleaf*)

SINUSITIS AND CATARRH (continued)

Aching in bones of face, worse in warm room and at night-time. Sneezing worse in sunshine. Nostrils feel raw, ulcerated, swollen. Yellowish green pus-like discharge.	**Mercurius Solubilis 6c.** One dose 4 times a day. Stop with improvement.
Bloodstained discharge. Severe pain in bones of face which are very sensitive to cold draughts. Generally worse at night and from cold air. Yellow, thick, ropy but fluid discharge from nose, and posterior nasal drip.	**Mezereum 6c** or **30c.** One dose 4 times a day. Stop with improvement.
Very offensive pus-like discharge. Throbbing, bursting pain. Restless. Fanlike motion of nostrils. Relief from motion and warmth.	**Pyrogen 6c** or **30c.** One dose morning and evening. Stop with improvement.
Catarrh headache before discharge appears. Fullness at root of nose; constant need to blow nose, but with no discharge. Worse for change of temperature.	**Sticta 6c.** One dose 4 times a day. Stop with improvement.

SKIN – OILY OR GREASY

Although greasy or oily skin tends to run in families, it is usually worse in adolescence, and is most obvious on the face. There is a tendency towards spots called blackheads and whiteheads, caused by the blocking of the sebaceous glands in the skin. These can become infected and the whole condition is called acne (see pages 106–7).

But greasy skin can also be found on the neck, across the shoulders and back, and on the central upper part of the chest, with or without spots.

The whole condition can be made worse by hormone imbalance, either naturally occurring in adolescence; before, during or after the menstrual periods; or by taking oral contraceptives.

External Treatment

- Avoid harsh chemical treatments and over-washing.
- Sunlight is helpful but avoid over exposure.
- Bathe with diluted solution of **Calendula** or **Hamamelis**.

Oily, sticky perspiration, smells unpleasant. Worse at night.	**Mercurius Solubilis 6c.** One dose morning and evening. Stop with improvement.
Face and forehead oily and shining. Dry crusting at skin margins and bends of joints.	**Natrum Muriaticum 6c.** One dose morning and evening. Stop with improvement.
Oily dirty-looking skin. Dry, lustreless, rough hair. Dreads cold draughts.	**Psorinum 6c.** One dose morning and evening. Stop with improvement.
Pimples, pustules and blind boils in shining skin.	**Selenium 6c.** One dose morning and evening. Stop with improvement.

SLEEPLESSNESS

It is a rare person who has never had one sleeplesss night. Most people take the occasional 'bad night' in their stride and usually have a good idea why it occurred – e.g. too much alcohol, a large heavy meal too late in the day, an exciting evening at the theatre or cinema or a disturbing programme on TV, overwork, angry arguments with the family or work colleagues, or a local pain like toothache. Even more obvious causes are noisy activities in the neighbourhood, or the weather. Whatever the background to the insomnia, and however long it has gone on, the following self-help techniques will always help and may even remove the need for any medication at all.

- Exercise – a daily brisk walk of 20 to 30 minutes, with or without a sporting activity, two or three times a week.
- Attention to diet, e.g. additive-free foods, particularly in the elderly; reducing the number of drinks of tea, coffee and alcohol, both in total during the day and particularly at night.
- Relaxation techniques, e.g.
  - Yoga
  - Autogenic training (AT)
  - Transcendental meditation (TM)
  - Hypnotherapy
  - Physical techniques – as taught by most physiotherapists.
- Acupuncture, acupressure and aromatherapy have all been used successfully by many people.
- Counselling for long-term personal problems at work or in the family.
- For great anxiety or anger and resentment, write an 'emotional diary' to get distressing feelings 'out of the system'.

What is more important is recurring insomnia, and in the worst case, insomnia every night.

- This frequently falls into a pattern, which can be matched to the pattern of a deep-acting 'constitutional remedy'. This is a remedy for the 'whole person', rather than the specific symptom he or she is suffering from.
- There are also remedies which will help most patients with a particular physical (e.g. pains – see 'Pain', pages 172–9), or emotional cause for their insomnia, e.g. repressed anger or guilt, or overeating late in the day.
- Lastly there are remedies which will help particular types of insomnia, e.g. alternating with daytime drowsiness, or occurring at a regular time.

SLEEPLESSNESS

Great anxiety, very restless to the point of being agitated. In and out of bed. Fears being alone and death. Irritable weakness. Thirsty. Worse after midnight. Especially in a chilly, fastidious person.

Arsenicum Album 30c. One dose to be taken every evening. Stop with improvement.

Anxious, frightening dreams. Restless, irritable, angry, intolerant of pain. One cheek red and hot, the other cheek pale and cold.

Chamomilla 30c. One dose to be taken every evening. Stop with improvement.

Greatly overtired with worry and overwork, especially nursing a sick relative. Nausea at smell of food. Severe weakness with lassitude. Oversensitive to pain, movement or noise.

Cocculus 30c. One dose to be taken every evening. Stop with improvement.

Nervous, intelligent, overreactive. Oversensitive to pleasurable activities and surprises. Optimism. Rush of ideas. Very acute hearing and sensitive to noise.

Coffea Cruda 30c. One dose to be taken every evening. Stop with improvement.

Particularly in illness of elderly. Insomnia at same time as somnolence. Sudden starts with fear. Nervous spasmodic cough, worse lying, better sitting up. Nightmares or dreams of a sexual nature. Wants to be naked. Jealous and suspicious.

Hyoscyamus 30c. One dose to be taken every evening. Stop with improvement.

Sensitive, mentally active, irritable and angry. Unable to switch off from business concerns.

Nux Vomica 30c. One dose to be taken every evening. Stop with improvement.

SORE THROAT
(INFECTED TONSILS, TONSILLITIS, PHARYNGITIS)

Sore throat may precede the common cold or influenza, or may be caused by a throat infection. Homoeopathic remedies used at the onset of a sore throat may prevent symptoms developing further. Prompt use of the correct remedy may avoid the need for antibiotics.

Sudden Onset

When it comes on suddenly, it is frequently the only complaint apart from a possible raised temperature. Do not forget the basic treatments of:

- Rest – in bed if necessary.
- Fluids – plenty of them.
- Soft, easily swallowed foods.
- In the case of young children particularly, tepid sponging to bring the temperature down to comfortable levels. For older children, a good method is to allow them to play with toys in the bath while it cools down slowly.

Slow Onset

The early symptoms will be of a much more general type and will be the main indications for choosing your homoeopathic remedy.

SORE THROAT (INFECTED TONSILS, TONSILLITIS, PHARYNGITIS)

Sudden Onset

Fever, throat burning, smarting, dry, tingling, bright red. Hurts to swallow.

Aconite 30c. One dose every two to three hours for 3–4 doses. If no improvement, move on to a different remedy.

Throat *red* and glossy, swallowing painful and may spread to the ears. Very hot, dry skin, red face.

Belladonna 6c. One dose every two to three hours and reduce with improvement.

Throat red and raw, sore and smarting. Tongue swollen and coated yellow, indented by teeth. Great salivation but thirsty. Breath smells.

Mercurius Solubilis 6c. One dose every two to three hours and reduce with improvement.

Dark red, sore, full feeling. Each swallow causes pain to ears. Difficulty swallowing even water. Neck muscles stiff.

Phytolacca 6c. One dose every two to three hours and reduce with improvement.

Slow Onset

Frequent sore throats. Slowly developing sore throat. Tonsils and glands in neck always enlarged.

Baryta Carbonica 6c. One dose three to four times a day for 5–10 days.

Comes on slowly in humid weather. Heavy head. Neck and shoulders sore. Aching back with shivers up and down. Not very thirsty.

Gelsemium 6c. One dose three to four times a day for 2–4 days.

Previous 'cold'. 'Fishbone' or 'crumb' sensation. Throat very sensitive to touch. Irritable and sensitive to draughts.

Hepar Sulphuris 6c. One dose three to four times a day for 2–4 days.

TOOTHACHE

What we usually call toothache may have many causes, but it is usually due to 'bad teeth', and for that the cure is to visit the dentist.

There are many types of pain and many factors, such as the location of the pain, how it is affected by hot or cold drinks or foods, and the effect of eating, pressure or touch.

If there is throbbing, swelling of the gum or face, a rise in temperature and a general feeling of being unwell, there is likely to be an infection. There may also be an abscess forming, described variously as a dental abscess, a root abscess or a gum boil. (See also 'Dental Abscess', pages 130–1.)

The list of possible remedies is much larger than shown here, but one among the selection on the page opposite may help you until the dentist can deal with the problem.

Note: Remember to use **Arnica 6c** with or without **Hypericum 6c** before and after dental treatment.

TOOTHACHE

Local throbbing pain of a gum boil, with much swelling of the face and mouth.	**Apis 6c.** One dose every hour. Reduce with improvement.
Painful local swelling near tooth. Stabbing pain to the ear. Teeth feel loose and tender. Thirst with increased salivation.	**Mercurius Solubilis 6c.** One dose every hour for 6–8 hours.

Apis 6c and Mercurius Solubilis 6c can be taken alternately every hour for several doses.

Stabbing, shooting pain; neuralgia. Brought on by ice cream or very cold winds, or iced drinks.	**Aconite 6c.** One dose every fifteen minutes for 6–8 doses.
Patient is intolerant, restless and peevish with the severe pain. Worse at night. Worse with warm food or drinks.	**Chamomilla 6c.** One dose every fifteen minutes for 6–8 doses.
Obvious bad teeth but no gum boil. Bad breath and bitter taste.	**Kreosotum 6c.** One dose every hour. Reduce with improvement.
Teeth extremely sensitive to touch and feel long. Profuse salivation.	**Plantago 6c.** One dose every fifteen minutes for 6–8 doses.
Pain – drawing and tearing. Teeth very sensitive to touch or cold air. Worse at night and after food. Cheek may be swollen and red. Patient irritable and resentful.	**Staphysagria 6c.** One dose every fifteen minutes for 6–8 doses.

TRAVEL SICKNESS AND JET LAG

Travel sickness is a distressing condition which affects many children and some adults. It may vary from simple nausea and headaches to profuse vomiting and collapse.

Anxiety and excitement may play a part in the cause of travel sickness, especially in children, and being confined to a stuffy enclosed space may also be an important factor. Some people find that the fumes of fuel and exhausts and the smell of food or tobacco smoke make matters worse. Most of all, it is the actual motion of the transport and the sensitivity of the patient to the particular type of motion which is the main cause.

Jet lag occurs when the body is having problems adjusting to a changed time schedule, following a rapid shift in the course of a journey through several time zones.

Prevention

Anxiety and excitement can be treated before the journey as soon as the symptoms show themselves, even if this is two or three days before.

One or two doses of the remedy either for anxiety or for travel sickness may be given in the hour before the journey starts.

Treatment

Maintain a flow of fresh air during the journey. Provide children with games to take their minds off unpleasant symptoms. Allow for frequent stops during car journeys.

Throughout the book I normally indicate the use of a single remedy. But this can be difficult to find, especially in confusing situations such as a journey. If you are in doubt about the remedy, alternate the two most likely ones when the symptoms begin to return.

TRAVEL SICKNESS AND JET LAG

Anxiety Before the Journey

(See also 'Anxiety', pages 108–9.)

Gelsemium 6c, Ignatia 6c, Argentum Nitricum 6c. One or two doses before, and one repeated during the journey.

Excitement in Children

Coffea Cruda 6c. One or two doses before, and one repeated during the journey.

The Journey

Nausea, vomiting, saliva increased. Metallic taste in mouth. Worse thinking of food; much worse on sight or smell of food. Giddiness, and must lie down. Improved by warmth.

Cocculus 6c. One or two doses before the journey and on the return of any symptoms during the journey.

Nausea with greatly increased saliva. Empty feeling relieved by food. Vomiting and giddiness worse with noise. Headache in the neck and back of head. Improved by closing eyes.

Petroleum 6c. One or two doses before, and one repeated during the journey.

Nausea, vomiting and giddiness. Very pale, cold sweats, fainting. Collapse. Worse with smell of tobacco smoke. Headache like a band around the head. Improved by cold.

Tabacum 6c. One or two doses before, and one repeated during the journey.

Jet Lag

Bruised, tired feeling. Bed feels too hard. Must lie down but can't get comfortable. Restless and oversensitive.

Arnica 30c. One dose during the flight. Continue 2–3 times a day as needed. Stop with improvement.

Loss of sleep. Prostration. Sensation of hollowness and weakness. Anxiety. Nausea and/or dizziness. Loss of appetite.

Cocculus 30c. One dose during the flight. Continue 2–3 times a day as needed. Stop with improvement.

VARICOSE ULCERS

This is a very troublesome and painful condition which affects women far more than men. Not only are the ulcers painful and frequently infected, but the legs are swollen. It usually occurs after the formation of varicose veins. These arise because of:

- A family tendency
- Constipation
- Childbirth
- Standing at work for long periods with little movement of the leg muscles and insufficient rest
- Neglect of the earlier stages

Basic Treatment

- Seek medical advice. If neglected, varicose ulcers can become chronic and will fail to heal. Pressure bandaging will probably be recommended and must be applied by a trained person.
- Rest as much as possible, with the legs raised above body level, to help drain fluids from the legs.
- Select an appropriate homoeopathic remedy from the list opposite to assist with the healing process.
- Bathe with a solution of **Calendula** tincture, 5ml (twenty drops) to 200ml (half a pint) of cool, previously boiled water. However, only do this if your nurse or doctor agrees.

VARICOSE ULCERS

Extensive varicose veins, ulcers secreting thick yellow pus. Hard raised edges, with swollen and purple surrounding skin. Legs painful hanging down.	**Calcium Fluoricum 6c.** One dose twice a day. Stop with improvement.
A bruised soreness of varicose veins and a stinging or pricking pain in ulcers. Worse with heat. Bruised-looking skin.	**Hamamelis 6c.** One dose twice a day. Stop with improvement.
Dry, deep ulcers with overhanging edges. Do not tend to spread. Red surrounding skin. Pain worse in cold weather.	**Kali Bichromicum 6c**. One twice a day. Stop with improvement.
Irregular edges. Base looks like raw flesh. Ulcers bleed easily. Very sensitive. Burning pains or splinter-like pains, worse from touch at night and in very cold and very hot weather.	**Nitric Acid 6c**. One dose twice a day. Stop with improvement.
Ulcer raised and swollen with jagged itching edges, yellow pus. Surrounding skin swollen and with brownish discolouration.	**Sulphur 6c.** One dose twice a day. Stop with improvement.

WARTS (VERRUCAS)

Warts are the result of a virus invading the skin. The cells of the skin multiply rapidly and cause raised lumps, which are usually painless. But on the sole of the foot the weight of the body presses the wart into the deeper layers of the skin and they become painful, flattened and horny (verrucas).

Warts are made up of cauliflower heads – sometimes called 'seeds' – and become obvious when they are broken by injury, when they bleed easily. Such open warts are contagious to the patient and others. Especially infectious are the condylomata warts in the hot moist areas of the body, for example, the groin and crutch regions.

Local treatment is not really necessary, but it often helps the patient psychologically to use a local application. This is particularly true in the case of children.

Normally acid or caustic preparations are prescribed, but they can both be dangerous and can cause scarring. Apply some **Thuja** mother tincture to the wart each evening using a cotton bud. Take by mouth the homoeopathic remedy that best matches the description.

WARTS (VERRUCAS)

Greasy dirty brown skin, freckles and blotches. Blackheads. Nails soft and flaking. Black warts on any part of body and scalp. Appearance of seeds in the wart. Condylomata in the genital area.

Thuja 6c. One dose morning and evening for several weeks.

(*Note:* Thuja is the main underlying remedy.)

Horny and hard warts on any part of the body but especially on the soles of the feet and the palms of the hands. Thickening and cracking of the soles and palms. Nails thick and hard, splitting lengthwise.

Antimonium Crudum 6c. One dose morning and evening for several weeks.

Flattened warts under the nails or on the end of the nose and upper eyelids. Also warts which are flat, hollowed out or tall and thin, but bleed easily.

Causticum 6c. One dose morning and evening for several weeks.

Small flat transparent warts on the back of the hands, better seen in reflected rather than direct light. Large dark fleshy warts on the backs of fat people.

Dulcamara 6c. One dose morning and evening for several weeks.

Hard yellow horny wart with yellow surrounding area of skin. Fissures which bleed; needle-like pain.

Nitric Acid 6c. One dose morning and evening for several weeks.

(This remedy may be used in conjunction with Antimonium Crudum – take Antimonium Crudum in the morning and Nitric Acid in the evening.)

Fleshy warty growths with severe itching, numbness and burning in genital area. Bleed easily. Constantly moist. Blackheads in the skin.

Sabina 6c. One dose morning and evening for several weeks.

(It may improve the treatment to add either one dose of **Thuja 30c** each week, or one dose of **Nitric Acid 6c** each day to the Sabina dosage.)

Warts on neck with 'horn' in centre. Small flat warts with itching; on face and hands. Dark, painless with 'seeds'.

Sepia 6c. One dose morning and evening for several weeks.

A Basic Materia Medica

In the first part of this book, the illness or injury itself is discussed, together with the different groups of symptoms that indicate which particular homoeopathic remedies are likely to be needed to treat the individual patients.

What follows in the next few pages is a list of homoeopathic remedies, together with a brief description of the diseases and conditions which might be helped by each one. Each description of a remedy involves the sorts of minor ailments that can reasonably be treated at home, and at the same time begins to build up a description of the 'properties' of the remedy.

The 'properties' or 'characteristics' of a remedy relate to the kind of physical and emotional symptoms that recur in any individual's life, and to the particular external and emotional circumstances that affect their well-being, either positively or adversely. It is found that amongst the major homoeopathic remedies there will be one which is of special value to the person who corresponds more or less to such a 'symptom picture'. The remedy is thus directly relevant to that individual's constitution, and such remedies are known as 'constitutional remedies'.

The short remedy pictures that follow are only outline descriptions of some of the important constitutional remedies in homoeopathy. If you wish to extend your knowledge of the remedies, especially the emotional and more general characteristics, there are several books which you might find helpful. Ask for advice on this from any of the organisations listed on pages 216 and 217. I have deliberately not gone into these aspects of the remedies in the brief sketches below, because I do not think it helps the particular purpose of this book, which is First Aid.

Aconite

SHOCK — CROUP — FRIGHT — FEVER — ACCIDENTS — CHILLS

The beginning of colds, flu, fevers – especially if restless, anxious, thirsty or severely chilled.

In emergencies like accidents, bereavements, animal or insect bites, asthma or bleeding, especially if distressed, with fear, palpitations of the heart, breathlessness, trembling and numbness and tingling of the face and fingers.

Antimonium Crudum

UPSET STOMACH

No appetite, with belching, bloated stomach, white thickly-coated tongue, cracked corners of the mouth.
Depressed and irritable. Baby vomits feeds.
Sick headaches from thick catarrh, too much alcohol, bathing.
Feels better with acid drinks or pickles.

Antimonium Tartaricum

COUGH

Wheezing bronchitis, rattling cough, difficult to get the phlegm up.
Breathless, suffocating, gasping, must sit up to get ease.
Pale-faced, weak, clammy cold skin.

Arnica

INJURY

If shocked, give Aconite first.
Bruising, sprains, concussion, accidents, operations.
Aching muscles from over-use in work or sports.
Before and after dental surgery (with Hypericum).
Overtiredness.

Arsenicum Album

VOMITING AND DIARRHOEA – FOOD POISONING – GASTRIC FLU

Especially when vomiting and diarrhoea occur together.
Very chilly, anxious, restless, weak.
Burning pains in the stomach. Thirst – likes warm drinks.
Nauseated by sight and smell of food.

Belladonna

HIGH FEVER — THROBBING — SORE THROAT — SUNSTROKE — HEADACHE — EARACHE — BOILS

Very red cheeks, pale around the lips.
Wide open eyes, wide open pupils.
Excited, perhaps delirious. Thirsty but won't drink during a fever.
Very hot, dry skin, perhaps a scarlet rash.

Bryonia

PAINS — BURSTING HEADACHE

Arthritis, pleurisy, migraine.
Pains worse from movement, breathing, warmth.
Pains better for lying still, pressure, cool.
The patient is *very* thirsty for cold drinks.

Cantharis

CYSTITIS — BURNS AND SCALDS — BLISTERS — GNAT BITES

Cystitis – scalding, burning urine which may be bloodstained, passed in drops. Pain before, during and after urination. Painful urging. Frequency.

Burns and scalds – pain eased with cold applications.

Carbo Vegetabilis

WIND — FLATULENCE — COLLAPSE

Stomach distended and belching wind. Relieved by sitting up and loosening clothes. General physical collapse with skin pale or bluish. Pulseless. Cold. Cold sweat. Gasping for fresh air and feels better if the face is fanned and propped up.

Chamomilla

UNBEARABLE PAIN. Frantic child with EARACHE, TOOTHACHE, TEETHING, COLIC

The child may be pacified by being picked up but may remain very difficult, irritable and angry. One cheek may be red and hot.
Generally may be made worse by bouts of anger.
Green diarrhoea may accompany the colic.

Colocynthis

COLIC — NEURALGIC PAIN — GRIPING PAIN

Three-month colic in babies.
Abdominal colic eased by bending over, firm pressure or a hot water bottle.
Griping pains distended with wind, belching, vomiting.
Colic or neuralgia from anger, resentment or becoming worked up.

Euphrasia

HAY FEVER — MEASLES

Measles, early stage with streaming tears that burn, photophobia (pain in the eyes from too much light). Head throbs.
Sneezing, running nose, cough.
Hay fever with similar symptoms, made worse indoors, in the evenings or in warm weather.

Gelsemium

INFLUENZA — HEADACHE — ANXIETY — SORE THROAT

Influenza – drowsy, 'drugged' feeling. Weakness.
Aching, shivery back.
Aching, trembling limbs.
'Thick head' – aching back of head, neck, heavy-eyed.
Sneezing, running nose, sore throat and painful swallowing. Not thirsty.
Anxiety – especially *before* an event or difficult situation.

Hepar Sulphuris

BOILS — ABSCESSES — INFECTED SPOTS — TONSILLITIS — COUGH

Tonsillitis with splinter-like pains (sometimes extending into the ear).
Cough dry and deep with tightness of the chest or cough with wheezing and rattling chest.
Patients can be irritable, oversensitive, discontented, grumbling and impetuous. They usually feel better in warm, wet weather, but their problems can be made worse by touch or cold draught.

Hypericum

WOUNDS OR OPERATIONS — PAINFUL INJURIES TO NERVES OF FINGERS, TOES, NAILS, LIPS, GUMS AND TEETH

Any sort of injury where the nerve endings have been damaged, causing severe pain and sensitivity.
Before and after dental treatment or operations.

Ipecacuanha

NAUSEA — COUGH

Continuous nausea with no relief from vomiting. Clean tongue and too much saliva.
Cough with congested, wheezing chest. Nosebleeds and other haemorrhages with nausea.

Mercurius Solubilis

FEVERISH COLDS — ULCERATED MOUTH AND THROAT

Offensive-smelling sweat, breath or mucus.
Generally weak and trembling.
Feels chilly in the cold, too hot in the warmth.
Greatly increased saliva but very thirsty.
Profuse yellow, green catarrh.
Diarrhoea persisting with painful straining, slime and perhaps blood.
Worse at night and in the warmth.

Natrum Muriaticum

SNEEZING — COLDS — COLD SORES

Profuse watery nasal catarrh with sneezing.
Generally chilly but worse in a warm room.
Greasy skin, likes salt, thirsty.
Weary, weepy and irritable. Effects of grief.

Nux Vomica

UPSET STOMACH — INDIGESTION — INFLUENZA — HEADACHE

Indigestion – from too much food or alcohol. Belching bitter fluid. Bloated 'heavy weight' feeling hours after eating. Hangover.
Nausea, constipation or frequent unsatisfactory bowel movements. Itching piles.
'Stuffy' cold with dry blocked nose, worse in the open air, improving in a warm room. Very irritable. Sensitive. Reproachful.

Influenza – with a very chilled feeling.

Phosphorus

LARYNGITIS — REPEATED VOMITING — BLEEDING

Nosebleeds. Bleeding after dental extractions.
Hoarse voice, painful talking, chest tight.
Loss of voice.
Cough – dry, tickling and racking, made worse by moving out into cold air and by talking.
Gastritis – wants cold drinks but soon vomits them back up.

Pulsatilla

CATARRH — MEASLES — INDIGESTION

Catarrh – yellow-green, in eyes or nose.
Loss of sense of smell.
Dry mouth but *not* thirsty.
Loose cough worse in a warm room.
Measles – catarrhal stage with a greenish-yellow nasal catarrh.
Indigestion from fatty, oily or rich foods.
Generally feels much better in fresh air.

Rhus Toxicodendron

ARTHRITIS — FIBROSITIS — RHEUMATISM — SHINGLES — SPRAINS

Pains and stiffness – worse in cold, wet weather, cold air, after rest, on getting up from a chair or out of bed.
First movements painful and stiff – keeping moving eases the pain and stiffness.
Influenza with rheumaticky pains and stiffness and a dry cough.
Itching, tender blisters and rash. Mouth ulcers and cold sores.

Sulphur

SKIN RASHES

Burning, itching skin rashes. Eczema.
Worse for heat of bed, scratching, bathing and clothes.
Boils, styes, piles – burning pain.
Morning diarrhoea.
To conclude treatment for infections and inflammations.

The Medicine Chest

The domestic 'medicine chest' for homoeopathic medicines is really a container for all the remedies which have accumulated over a period of time. It can be any convenient box or tin. In contrast to ordinary medicines, it is quite safe to keep homoeopathic remedies for future use.

Some homoeopathic pharmacists still dispense remedies in the traditional 7 gram glass tubes and sell boxes containing compartments for each tube. Others dispense in either glass or plastic containers of differing sizes. It is useful to write the names of the remedy and the potency on a circular label on the plastic screw top. Another useful tip is to print a sheet of card in the top of the box as an alphabetical list of each remedy with the potency.

A basic list of remedies follows, together with an extended list.

As you treat yourself and the family you will obtain a variety of remedies, and some tablets or pills will be left over. Do not throw them away, but keep them to build up your medicine chest. They will reflect the common problems of your family and will be readily to hand if needed.

BASIC LIST OF HOMOEOPATHIC REMEDIES FOR STARTING THE MEDICINE CHEST

Aconite
Antimonium Crudum
Antimonium Tartaricum
Arnica
Arsenicum Album
Belladonna
Bryonia
Chamomilla
Ipecacuanha
Mercurius Solubilis
Natrum Muriaticum
Nux Vomica
Phosphorus

Plus: Hypercal tincture, and Arnica and Rhus Tox. creams

EXTENDED LIST OF HOMOEOPATHIC REMEDIES

Allium Cepa
Apis
Argentum Nitricum
Cantharis
Carbo Vegetabilis
Cocculus
Colocynthis
Drosera
Euphrasia
Ferrum Phosphoricum
Gelsemium
Hamamelis
Hepar Sulphuris
Hypericum
Ignatia
Ledum
Lycopodium
Pulsatilla
Rhus Toxicodendron
Ruta
Sepia
Spongia
Sulphur
Urtica Urens

SOME HOMOEOPATHIC OINTMENTS AND CREAMS

Aesculus Hippocastanum – swollen, prolapsing piles.

Arnica – for bruising (but *not* with broken skin).

Calendula – for cuts and grazes; antiseptic effect. Stimulates the healing process.

Graphites – skin problems, especially when broken and oozing clear fluid.

Hamamelis – for bruising with broken skin; bleeding piles.

Hypericum – crushed nerve endings; bed sores. Can be made up in a bland oil.

Paeonia – unbearable itching: piles and anus, vulva, skin.

Rhus Toxicodendron – joints which are stiff in cold, damp weather.

Ruta – sprains and strains; internal damage.

Tamus – chilblains.

Urtica Urens – burns and sunburn; stinging eczema; itching vulva; nettle rash (urticaria).

TINCTURES

Arnica – for bruising.

Calendula – for grazes and wounds.

'Hypercal' – for grazes and wounds. This is a mixture of the tinctures of Hypericum and Calendula.

Urtica Urens – for burns or itching.

The First Aid Box

It is useful and more efficient to have First Aid items together in a suitably marked box which is always kept in the same place. Personal preference plays a large part in what you have in it, but the following list may be a useful guide to begin with:

1) Adhesive plasters, assorted sizes.
2) Adhesive plaster, one roll. (Remember that some people may be allergic to certain types of plaster. Ask the pharmacist for advice on what to get.)
3) Cotton wool, one sterilised small pack.
4) Wound dressing, sterilised and *non*-medicated. Small, medium and large, two of each.
5) Gauze squares, sterilised and *non*-medicated, one pack.
6) Gauze bandages, sterilised and *non*-medicated, assorted sizes.
7) Eye pad, sterilised and with tapes.
8) Crepe bandage, 8cm wide.
9) Small round-ended scissors.
10) Tweezers for applying dressings.

Organisations Concerned With Homoeopathy

The Faculty of Homoeopathy

Membership of the Faculty is only open to doctors medically qualified in the United Kingdom or in countries and medical schools recognised by the General Medical Council. Members and Fellows have all received postgraduate training in homoeopathic medicine and passed the examination of the Faculty. They use the letters MFHom or FFHom after their other qualifications. For names and addresses of such doctors in the UK and worldwide, contact: The Faculty of Homoeopathy, Royal London Homoeopathic Hospital, Great Ormond Street, London WC1N 3HR. Tel: 0171–837–9469, Fax: 0171–278–7900.

Homoeopathic Hospitals within the UK National Health Service

Any general practitioner working within the UK National Health Service is able to refer his or her patients to the following NHS hospitals for an appointment with a consultant homoeopathic physician:

Bristol Homoeopathic Hospital, Cotham Hill, Bristol BS6 6JU.
Tel: 0117-973-1231, Fax: 0117-923-8759

Glasgow Homoeopathic Hospital, 1000 Great Western Road, Glasgow G12 0NR. Tel: 0141–334–9800, Fax: 0141–211–1610

Baillieston Homoeopathic Outpatients Clinic, 62 Buchanan Street, Glasgow G69 7AD. Tel: 0141-771-7396

Mossley Hill Hospital, Park Avenue, Liverpool L18 8BU.
Tel: 0151–250–3000, Fax: 0151–729–0191

Royal London Homoeopathic Hospital, Great Ormond Street, London WC1N 3HR. Tel: 0171–837–9469, Fax: 0171–278–7900

Tunbridge Wells Homoeopathic Hospital, Church Road, Tunbridge Wells TN1 1JU. Tel: 01892-542977

(*continued overleaf*)

Further Information

The following organisations can supply information on where homoeopathic treatment may be obtained, as well as the addresses of local suppliers of homoeopathic remedies. Many of them produce publications in the subject at various levels, and some also stock recommended books on homoeopathy for retail sale, generally by post.

UK

British Homoeopathic Association, 27a Devonshire Street, London W1N 1RJ. Tel: 0171–935–2163, Fax: 0171–486–2957

The Homoeopathic Society, 2 Powis Place, Great Ormond Street, London WC1N 3HT. Tel: 0171–837–9469, Fax: 0171–278–7900

Natural Medicines Society, Market Chambers, 13a Market Place, Heanor DE75 5AA. Tel. 01773–710002

USA

American Board of Homeotherapeutics (same as National Center for Homeopathy, below)

American Institute of Homeopathy, 925 East 17th Avenue, Denver, CO 80218. Tel: (303) 861–4181

Council for Homeopathic Certification, 1709 Seabright Avenue, Santa Cruz, CA 95062. Tel: (408) 421–0565

Homeopathic Academy of Naturopathic Physicians, 11231 S.E. Market Street, Portland, OR 97216. Tel: (503) 795–0579

Homeopathic Educational Services, 2124 Kittredge Street, Berkeley, CA 94704. Tel: (510) 649–0294, Fax: (510) 649–1955

International Foundation for Homeopathy, P.O. Box 7, Edmonds, WA 98020. Tel: (206) 776–4147, Fax: (206) 776–1499

National Center for Homeopathy, 801 North Fairfax, Suite 306, Alexandria, VA 22314. Tel: (703) 548–7790, Fax: (703) 548–7792

Professional (non-medical) homoeopaths

In addition to homoeopathic doctors, there are also trained professional homoeopathic practitioners who are not medically qualified. The Society of Homoeopaths maintains a register of those practitioners whom it recognises as being qualified and competent to practice. The Society is in communication with other societies of professional homoeopaths outside the UK and can supply information on similar organisations worldwide. For further details, contact: The Society of Homoeopaths, 2 Artizan Road, Northampton NN1 4HU. Tel: 01604–21400, Fax: 01604–22622.

Major Suppliers of Homoeopathic Remedies (partial list)

Ainsworths Homoeopathic Pharmacy, 36 New Cavendish Street, London W1M 7LH, UK

Biological Homeopathic Industries, 11600 Cochiti S.E., Albuquerque, NM 87123, USA

Boericke and Tafel, 2381 Circadian Way, Santa Rosa, CA 95407, USA

Boiron USA, 6 Campus Boulevard, Bldg A, Newtown Square, PA 19073, USA

Brauer Biotherapies, P.O. Box 234, Tanunda 5352, Australia

Dolisos USA, 3014 Rigel Avenue, Las Vegas, NV 89102, USA

Helios Homoeopathic Pharmacy, 92 Camden Road, Tunbridge Wells TN1 2QP, UK

Nelson's Homoeopathic Pharmacy, 15 Duke Street, Dublin 2, Ireland

Nelson's Homoeopathic Pharmacy, 73 Duke Street, London W1M 6BY, UK

Standard Homeopathic Co., 210 West 131st Street, Los Angeles, CA 90061, USA

Thompsons Homeopathic Supplies, 844 Yonge Street, Toronto, Ont. M4W 2H1, Canada

Weleda Ireland, Sroughan, Lacken, Blessington, Co. Wicklow, Ireland

Weleda NZ, P.O. 8132, Te Mata Peak Road, Havelock North, New Zealand

Weleda SA, P.O. 5502, Johannesburg 2000, South Africa

Weleda UK, Heanor Road, Ilkeston, Derbyshire DE7 8DR, UK

Weleda USA, P.O. Box 249, Congers, NY 10920, USA

Important Telephone Numbers

General Practitioner:

Homoeopath:

Dentist:

District Nurse:

Midwife:

Health Visitor:

Ambulance – *in emergency only* – Dial 999 or 112

Homoeopathic Pharmacy:

Acupuncturist:

Chiropractor:

Osteopath:

Others:

INDEX OF REMEDIES

INDEX OF PROBLEMS

Classical Homoeopathy, Dr Margery Blackie, 1986, reprinted 1990 with Repertory. The complete teaching legacy of one of the most important homoeopaths of our time. 0906584140

Comparative Materia Medica, Dr E. F. Candegabe, 1997. Detailed comparative study of thirty-seven remedies. 0906584361

Homoeopathic Prescribing, Dr Noel Pratt, revised 1985. A compact reference book covering 161 common complaints and disorders, with guidance on the choice of the appropriate remedy. 0906584035

Homoeopathic Treatment of Beef and Dairy Cattle, The, C. E. I. Day, MRCVS, FFVetHom, 1995. Describes how homoeopathy may be used in the care of cattle, both as individuals and in a group. 090658437X

Homoeopathic Treatment of Eczema, The, Robin Logan, FSHom, 1997. A textbook on the homoeopathic treatment of this condition. 0906584477

Homoeopathy, Dr T. P. Paschero (in translation). Dr Paschero's major work on the subject. 0906584418

Homoeopathy as Art and Science, Dr Elizabeth Wright Hubbard, 1990. The selected writings of one of the foremost modern homoeopaths. 0906584264

Homoeopathy in Practice, Dr Douglas Borland, 1982, reprinted 1988 with Symptom Index. Detailed guidance on the observation of symptoms and the choice of remedies. 090658406X

In Search of the Later Hahnemann, Rima Handley MA, DPhil, FSHom, 1997. A study of Hahnemann's practice in Paris, with material from his casebooks of that period. 0906584353

Insights into Homoeopathy, Dr Frank Bodman, 1990. Homoeopathic approaches to common problems in general medicine and psychiatry. 0906584280

Introduction to Homoeopathic Medicine (2nd Edition), Dr Hamish Boyd, 1989. A formal introductory text, written in categories that are familiar to the medical practitioner. 0906584213

Materia Medica of New Homoeopathic Remedies, Dr O. A. Julian, paperback edition 1984. Full clinical coverage of 106 new homoeopathic remedies, for use in conjunction with the classical materia medicas. 0906584116

Other Books in the Beaconsfield Homoeopathic Library

Mental Symptoms in Homoeopathy, Dr Luis Detinis, 1994. A comparative study of the Mind rubrics in Kent's *Repertory*. 0906584345

Studies of Homoeopathic Remedies, Dr Douglas Gibson, 1987. Detailed clinical studies of 100 major remedies. Well-known for the uniquely wide range of insights brought to bear on each remedy. 0906584175

Tutorials on Homoeopathy, Dr Donald Foubister, 1989. Detailed studies on a wide range of conditions and remedies. 0906584256

Typology in Homoeopathy, Dr Léon Vannier, 1992. A study of human types, based on the gods of Antiquity, and the remedies which are relevant to them. 0906584302

– NOTES –

– NOTES –

– NOTES –

– NOTES –

– NOTES –